Proceedings of the Eighth Annual Conference of the British Association for Biological Anthropology and Osteoarchaeology

Edited by

Megan Brickley
Martin Smith

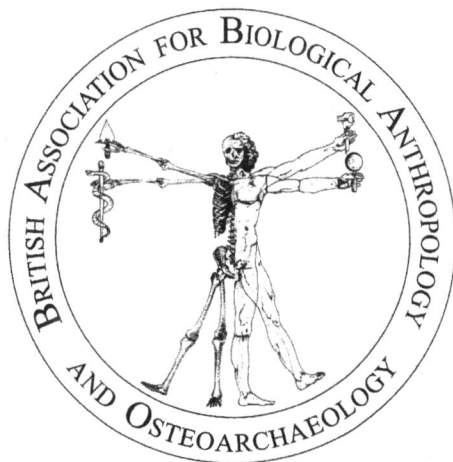

BAR International Series 1743
2008

Published in 2016 by
BAR Publishing, Oxford

BAR International Series 1743

*Proceedings of the Eighth Annual Conference of the British Association for Biological
Anthropology and Osteoarchaeology*

ISBN 978 1 4073 0185 3

BAR Publishing is the trading name of British Archaeological Reports (Oxford) Ltd.
British Archaeological Reports was first incorporated in 1974 to publish the BAR
Series, International and British. In 1992 Hadrian Books Ltd became part of the BAR
group. This volume was originally published by Archaeopress in conjunction with
British Archaeological Reports (Oxford) Ltd / Hadrian Books Ltd, the Series principal
publisher, in 2008. This present volume is published by BAR Publishing, 2016.

Printed in England

BAR

PUBLISHING

BAR titles are available from:

BAR Publishing
122 Banbury Rd, Oxford, OX2 7BP, UK
EMAIL   info@barpublishing.com
PHONE   +44 (0)1865 310431
FAX   +44 (0)1865 316916
www.barpublishing.com

Contents

Introduction

Martin Smith and Megan Brickley

Institute of Archaeology and Antiquity, University of Birmingham,
Edgbaston, Birmingham, B15 2TT

This volume presents the fourth publication of papers presented at an annual meeting of the British Association for Biological Anthropology and Osteoarchaeology (BABAO). The papers contained here are a sample of those given at the eighth annual meeting of BABAO, held at the University of Birmingham between 15th and 17th September 2006. The conference was attended by 110 delegates from seven countries in addition to the UK, with the association continuing to promote and encourage development within the field of biological anthropology. The studies presented here have been subject to full peer-review.

As at previous BABAO meetings the conference programme included a diverse and varied selection of presentations that provide a snapshot of the breadth of contrasting methods, periods and questions being approached within the discipline. Papers in this volume cover periods ranging from Anglo Saxon times to the high Middle Ages and onwards up to the early 20th century. Whilst some chapters focus on specific skeletal samples, others are more methodological with the subjects covered including aspects as diverse as anthropometrics, palaeopathology, the history and development of medicine, identifying immigration in archaeological populations and modern forensics. The studies included are also geographically varied, ranging in latitude from Tierra Del Fuego to Sweden, with those in between including New Guinea, Palestine and France as well as studies covering various parts of Britain. The contents of this volume differ additionally in terms of scale from the level of individual case studies to work investigating events which affected the lives of thousands.

The initial session of the conference entitled 'Written in Bone' presented work involving the use of written sources in investigating health and disease in the past. Despite the specific nature of this theme the papers presented were broad ranging both in the questions addressed and the approaches taken. The two keynote speakers Ann Herring and Piers Mitchell were funded by a grant from the Wellcome trust. Ann Herring[*] presents an important and interesting study of the 1918 influenza pandemic which uses military documentation from the time to infer the location of the initial outbreak of the infection. The resultant conclusions differ from views derived from secondary sources and also from that given in the official War Record, underlining the importance of using multiple lines of evidence to investigate past health and disease. Piers Mitchell uses evidence for ill-health and medical treatment during the crusades to illustrate the benefits of combining skeletal data with both contemporary written sources and other categories of archaeological evidence. In particular he advocates the greater use by physical anthropologists of written sources in their original languages in order to avoid the multi-layered problems of interpretation that may result when only using sources in translation or when enlisting a third party to extract information from contemporary documents.

Continuing the theme of the development of medicine Amna Suliman and Lisa Brent's chapters present investigations of 19th century medical practice which combine written records from the time with data derived from skeletal specimens curated by the Imperial College London Pathology Museum. The former uses a specific case study to explore the changing social and medical attitudes towards women and illness (specifically tuberculosis) and the role played by emerging technologies in changing such ideas. Conversely, Lisa Brent's chapter focuses on the protracted failure of physicians to effectively treat rickets prior to the 1880s in spite of the rapid advances that had occurred with regard to treating many arguably more complex conditions. Caroline Arcini's chapter presents emerging data obtained during analysis of an 18th and 19th century cemetery assemblage from Sweden and outlines some of the problems and prospects surrounding attempts to identify the remains of specific individuals from contemporary documents. Closer to home Jacqueline McKinley presents a detailed study of an 18th century Quaker community from Dorset. This investigation revealed unexpected insights regarding the demographic make-up of the population which are discussed in light of religious, economic and geographic factors which may have been responsible. This work is of further significance as despite the recent growth of studies on post-medieval cemetery assemblages, few osteological analyses have so far been published in relation to provincial populations. Discussion following the session, which is exemplified by the papers published in this volume, served to illustrate the way in which a wider perspective can be gained on past populations when historical and archaeological sources are combined. With increased analysis of sites from periods with text based evidence, particularly the very recent past, this approach will hopefully be increasingly adopted.

As always the meeting's Open session drew a particularly diverse range of presentations. Charlotte Henderson's work on enthesopathies studies the relationship between bone-forming diseases and bony changes more usually associated

---

[*] NB Some papers are multiply authored, see contents page/ chapters for full compliment of authors.

with musculo-skeletal stress, concluding that individuals suffering from these conditions need to be excluded from a given sample before conclusions can be drawn about such activity related skeletal changes. Focusing on a single condition, Paola Ponce explores the possible connection between the development of bony anomalies surrounding the external auricular canal and exposure to cold water at extremes of latitude by examining two skeletal samples from southern Chile. In a more methodological vein Alan Ogden's paper provides a clear and logical guide to the identification and recording of voids in human jaw bones. This is an area previously fraught with misdiagnosis and in need of clarification. Consequently this paper constitutes an important contribution to the literature that is likely to be of use to a wide range of researchers. Using a cemetery population from Anglo-Saxon Essex, Sarah Inskip provides a practical account of the issues and challenges involved in re-organising and re-cataloguing previously excavated skeletal collections, highlighting a useful sample with good future research potential in the process. Finally, Lisa Cashmore uses a sample from Papua New Guinea to explore the relative usefulness of two different skeletal measurements as predictors of body mass using a morphometric approach in contrast to more traditional biomechanical methods.

Two contributions are also included from the remaining conference sessions the first of which focused upon studies of movement and migration in which Natasha Powers' chapter discusses the potential for identifying both the impact of immigration and the physical remains of immigrants themselves within a cemetery population from 19th century London. The final session focused on studies of skeletal samples which reveal evidence of violence and conflict. This is an area previously somewhat neglected by archaeologists that has received increasing attention during recent years with a wide range of publications appearing on the subject. However, whilst many such studies have made frequent use of data derived from human remains, there had not previously been a conference session on this subject organised specifically by physical anthropologists. Catherine Tennick's paper drew the conference neatly to a close by presenting an experimental study of cut marks which applies criteria used to study incision marks made on bone with prehistoric tools to analyse marks made with modern metal implements. As such this work is likely to interest both modern forensic researchers and those investigating past evidence for violence on the skeleton.

Human remains constitute the most direct source of evidence available for investigating the lives of past communities and individuals. At a time when calls are coming from some quarters for archaeological collections of human remains to be reburied, these studies and others that continue to be published by BABAO members (www.babao.org.uk) illustrate the value of scientific work conducted within the field of biological anthropology which frequently provides new information and addresses questions which are not accessible using other types of evidence. The range and diversity of the studies presented here further underline the continuing need for an association like BABAO to bring researchers together and provide a forum for the exchange and publication of ideas in order for biological anthropology in Britain to continue to flourish and diversify in the future. We would like to thank all the authors whose work is presented here and we are also very grateful to all the referees who gave their time and expertise in reviewing the papers presented and without whom this volume would not have been possible.

Martin Smith and Megan Brickley

The geographical epicentre of the 1918 influenza pandemic

D. Ann Herring* and Janet Padiak

Department of Anthropology, McMaster University, Hamilton, Ontario, L8S 4L9, Canada
*e-mail address for correspondence: herring@mcmaster.ca

Abstract

There continues to be debate about the geographical origins of the 1918 influenza pandemic, fuelled by documentary evidence and PCR analysis of tissue samples drawn from individuals who died during the pandemic. Proponents of a European origin argue that the lethal virus was pre-seeded among British troops on the continent prior to 1918. The hypothesis is based primarily on secondary sources that describe pre-1918 cases of purulent bronchitis among British soldiers. The symptoms are judged to be indistinguishable from those described for the 1918 strain of influenza while conditions at army bases fostered the emergence of an epidemic. We address the pre-seeding hypothesis using primary source data from surviving British War Diaries kept by medical personnel during World War I. The Diaries depict all illnesses, not just cases admitted to hospital. They show that influenza outbreaks were sporadic and limited prior to 1918. Influenza seems to have been a relatively small problem compared to sexually transmitted diseases, dysentery, and diarrhoea. Soldiers ill with influenza in the spring of 1918 were felled again by the lethal strain circulating during autumn that year, which suggests that the strain of influenza during the first wave provided little protection against the second. The documentary and biological evidence for the 1918 pandemic reveals a complex and equivocal picture, underlining the importance of using multiple lines of evidence to study disease in the past.

Keywords: purulent bronchitis; Spanish Flu; British War Diaries; British Expeditionary Forces

Introduction

The combined use of documents and biological remains to address questions in human history offers the chance to approach questions of interest from multiple points of view, taking advantage of the different types of information and methodologies that come from each perspective. This is certainly true of research on the 1918 influenza pandemic where it has been possible to resurrect the genome of the H1N1 virus from archived human remains (Reid *et al.,* 1999; Taubenberger *et al,.* 2005) and to explore some of the questions that remain unsolved, such as why it was so lethal (Kobasa *et al,.* 2007), within the context of recorded accounts and statistics from the period.

Despite this wealth of information, there are still issues that remain to be clarified, such as the origins of the deadly pandemic, which is the subject of this paper. Although "[i]t is probable that it will never be definitely settled where the severe and fatal form of influenza arose in the fall of 1918" (Hall, 1928: 136), the U.S.A. and western Europe are currently the main contenders for this dubious honour. Our aim is not to resolve this debate. Rather, we present new information on the occurrence of influenza from 1916 to 1918 among British Expeditionary Forces in France. We suggest that this evidence undermines several of the fundamental principles of the European hypothesis as it is currently framed.

The epicentre problem

It is useful to review the basic arguments for the two leading locations for the epicentre of the 1918 influenza pandemic: Kansas, U.S.A. and northwest France.

American origins

Most authorities agree that the 1918 influenza pandemic began in the U.S.A. Proponents of an American origin argue from documentary evidence that the virus responsible for the pandemic emerged in the mid-west state of Kansas in the U.S.A. Military records show that in early March 1918 influenza struck soldiers at Camp Funston (now Fort Riley), Kansas (Crosby, 1989: 19). That month, there were 2840 cases of uncomplicated influenza from which everyone recovered. However, there were 56 deaths among the 3773 soldiers who suffered from complications of influenza, resulting in a death rate of 21.84 per 1000 (U.S. Surgeon General 1919). By the end of March, over 1900 recruits were sufficiently ill to require hospitalization (Hall, 1928: 133).

Swine influenza also appeared as a new disease in the U.S. mid-west around this time. John M. Barry (2004a: 92), historian and author of "The Great Influenza: The Epic Story of the 1918 Pandemic", suggests that a virulent virus had already emerged in Haskell County, Kansas – a sparsely populated county some 300 miles west of Camp Funston. Haskell County was farm country where people grew grain and raised poultry, cattle, and hogs. Any time ecological conditions create the opportunity for bird viruses to enter pigs, recombine with swine influenza viruses, and then infect humans, the conditions are ripe for the emergence of a new strain of influenza (Scholtissek, 1992, 1994).

In late January and early February of 1918, locals were "being struck down [by influenza] as suddenly as if they had been shot" (Barry, 2004b: 2). Barry claims this is the "first recorded instance suggesting that a new virus was adapting, violently, to man (sic)" (2004b: 3). He argues that recruits from Haskell County brought the virus with them to Camp Funston. Whatever the actual point of origin, army and civilian records show influenza jumping from army camp to army camp, then to cities, such as New York. Routinely collected death certificates and statistics show that an early wave of influenza and/or pneumonia was killing larger than expected numbers of New Yorkers from February to April 1918 (Olson, *et al.* 2005). New York was the port of embarkation of the American Expeditionary Force to the Western Front. Some 250,000 American soldiers sailed to Europe each month and hundreds of thousands were in U.S. training camps. Certainly there were reports of influenza deaths among the 15th U.S. Cavalry during their March voyage to Europe (Crosby, 1989: 25).

The emergence of influenza in Europe was closely tied to the arrival of American troops in France in the spring of 1918. Influenza was first reported in early April among the American Expeditionary Forces at Brest and in a rest camp near Bordeaux (Burnet and Clark, 1942: 70-71). It appeared later amongst other armies in France, suggesting to epidemiologists of the period that the ancestral virus had been brought to Europe by American soldiers (Patterson and Pyle, 1991: 8).

European origins

The idea of a European epicentre was explored but dismissed by distinguished scientists and epidemiologists who lived through the pandemic and studied its features, such as Australian Nobel laureate MacFarlane Burnet (Burnet and Clark, 1942) and Edwin Jordan (1927), who was commissioned by the American Medical Association to investigate the pandemic. The idea was revived several years ago by a British team headed by John Oxford, an eminent virologist at University College London (Oxford *et al.,* 2002, 2005). The argument draws attention to articles published from 1915 to 1917 in medical journals, such as *The Lancet*, that describe epidemics of 'purulent bronchitis' among British soldiers stationed at Aldershot, U.K. and Étaples, France, which suggests that the deadly virus was 'pre-seeded' in Europe prior to 1918 (c.f.: Hammond *et al.,* 1917).

The term 'purulent bronchitis' refers to the observation on autopsy of 'worms' of yellow pus oozing from the bronchioles of the lung. The symptoms and other clinical features of the 1915 to 1917 outbreaks are considered to be indistinguishable from the characteristic symptoms of influenza reported in 1918. In fact in 1919, Abrahams and colleagues (1919: 112) retrospectively described the 1917 epidemic at Aldershot as fundamentally the same as the 1918 outbreak. From these observations, together with a phylogenetic reconstruction of the virus that suggests that animal genes were introduced to Human Influenza A shortly before the 1918 pandemic, Oxford and colleagues propose that as much as two years earlier, a new virulent influenza virus may have been present among British troops.

The French town of Étaples figures prominently in the idea that virulent influenza was pre-seeded in Europe. Conditions present there before the 1918 outbreak are considered to be precisely those that would have allowed a new virus to evolve and spread quickly thereafter. Located on the northwest coast of France, Étaples was a large, over-crowded base for the British Expeditionary Force. From 1916 to 1918, it housed 100,000 soldiers on any given day and was a point of disembarkation for about 1 million soldiers en route to the Western Front. Here, battle-weary young men were brought together with fresh, epidemiologically naïve, new recruits. Military personnel lived in an environment contaminated with 23 gases, including chlorine, phosgene, and mustard gas (dichlorethyl sulphide), a known mutagen. Some 24 hospitals were tightly packed along the camp fringe, treating up to 23,000 men and women at any given time. A British army experiment introduced pig farms into the camp; there is photographic evidence for the presence of ducks, geese and chickens, and of soldiers purchasing and plucking them. In other words, "the conjunction of soldiers, gas, pigs, ducks, geese and horses in Northern France...provided the conditions" for "the rapid 'passage' of influenza in young soldiers", facilitating "small, step-wise mutational changes throughout the viral genome" (Oxford *et al.*, 2002: 113) that allowed an avian influenza virus to adapt to humans (Oxford *et al,.* 2005: 943).

The hypothesis suggests that military traffic from Europe to the U.S.A during 1917, as it prepared to enter the war, would have introduced the pathogen to the Americas. This would explain not only the early outbreaks in army camps in the U.S.A., but also a herald wave of influenza detected in New York City in 1917-1918 (c.f.: Olson *et al.,* 2005).

The British War Diaries

One of the weaknesses of the European epicentre hypothesis is that it rests on secondary sources: published accounts of unusual influenza outbreaks amongst troops in Britain and France prior to 1918. As anthropologists who work with archival information, we are interested in original documents created around the time of the pandemic, written about the daily life of ordinary rank and file soldiers. One of us (Padiak) has extensive experience studying British army records. We knew that the systematic collection of morbidity and mortality data on the soldiers went back a century, to the end of the Napoleonic wars (1815). If a virulent, influenza-like infection were present among British troops as early as 1916, then there should be evidence of some infectious disease, labelled as influenza or otherwise, among the daily records of the British Expeditionary Forces (BEF) stationed in France.

Our research is based on accounts and statistics contained in surviving British War Diaries (BWD) and Medical Services files from World War I, housed in the National Archives of the U.K., in Richmond, Surrey. These records are publicly available today but, as confidential documents, were withheld and not available for analysis before World War II. The British War Diaries provide weekly counts of morbidity, by disease, for each military unit of the British Expeditionary Forces.

In February 2005, Padiak collected photographs of the War Diaries for British and Canadian Expeditionary Forces from all five armies in France and Flanders from 1916 to 1918 (BEF HQ 1916-1918). The War diaries are organised on the same hierarchal basis as that of the entire expeditionary force. We consulted the diaries of the First and Second Armies, as well as divisions of the First Army, such as the Second Canadian Division. Valuable information was located in the war diaries of the Director General, Medical Services, of the British Expeditionary Force of France and Flanders, which oversaw the five armies of the BEF. We also perused the diaries of the British Force in the Forward Area in Italy. The bulk of the files used in this study is labelled as such: British Expeditionary Force, France and Flanders, General Headquarters, Director General, Medical Services, and then the year. We also consulted the reports of the BEF general headquarters for France and Flanders, casualty clearing units and lines of communication stations. The information on morbidity gleaned from these files was compiled in Microsoft Excel© spreadsheets, with separate spreadsheets for each division. Altogether the BWD data cover a force of some 1.9 million men, exclusive of officers. About 1.4 million were British and the remainder consisted of other nationalities such as Canadians, Australians and New Zealanders.

The Diaries are not personal accounts but official documents that record the military, sanitary and medical operations of each unit. Usually written by junior officers in pencil, or typed on onionskin paper, the Diaries also provide details on injuries, diseases and deaths, as well as precautions taken to prevent conditions that might foster disease transmission. Directives and reports are often appended to them. In effect, the Diaries document the everyday experience of medical people who lived through the war and treated the soldiers on a daily basis. The amount and type of information varies, depending on the size and scope of the military unit, where it stood in the military hierarchy, and the volubility of the individual keeping the Diary.

Some daily reports are several pages long, while others are relatively short, such as the sample excerpt below, written by the Assistant Director Medical Services 2nd Canadian Division, on February 15th 1916. This Division was located in the vicinity of Arras, France, about 30 km east of Étaples.

> "Feb 15th 1916 …Capt. H. B. J… of No 3 Field Ambulance improving, sputum negative to TB, temp moderate and now remaining nearly normal. Seems to have been one of several cases of a type of

bronchitis new to me, probably streptococcal in the main after a preliminary influenza infection, but in which the local signs of bronchitis are very slow in developing, and even more slow in subsiding. Convalescence in this climate and at this season is almost impossible. Three of the cases I have seen were Medical Officers, Lt-Col J…, Lieut N… RAMC (Temporary) of 18th Bde RGA and Capt H.B. J… There has been a moderate increase in respiratory disease in the division in the past week or so. (CWD 1915-8: Feb 15 1918)"

The excerpt exemplifies the quality and level of detail on infectious disease contained in the daily entries.

That said, the BWD sources present many challenges. The combination of pencil, flimsy paper, tiny writing because of wartime paper shortages, coupled with difficult field conditions, make many reports difficult if not impossible to read let alone photograph. Furthermore, there are gaps in reporting because of the exigencies of war. In many cases forces were disbanded and their members used to reinforce other units, resulting in a sudden cessation in a unit's Diaries. Reports may be complete for several months, missing for a month or two, and then resume. Some Diaries lack appendices. For example, the appendices with reports on infectious diseases were missing from the 2nd Canadian divisions for October 1918. This omission occurred after the final offensive and armistice and likely results from faulty file keeping.

Despite the patchiness of the British War Diary information, it has been possible to build a profile of the infectious disease load sustained by the British Expeditionary Forces. For the purposes of this paper, we focus on information from November 1916 to December 1918 gleaned from War Diaries for BEF troops in the vicinity of Arras, Calais, and Étaples in northern France and from Marseilles in southern France. This discussion is based on legible, typed reports that we acknowledge biases the information toward larger units with more permanent facilities.

The study period encompasses the mild, spring outbreak and lethal autumn outbreak of influenza in 1918. It also covers the pre-1918 influenza outbreaks of 'purulent bronchitis' published in medical journals. We are not aware of other studies that have used the War Diaries to examine questions about the 1918 influenza pandemic.

Recognizing influenza

Another challenge presented by this research was recognizing cases of influenza in the BWD records; some BEF reporters used the term, others didn't. This may seem odd, given that the term 'influenza' has been used

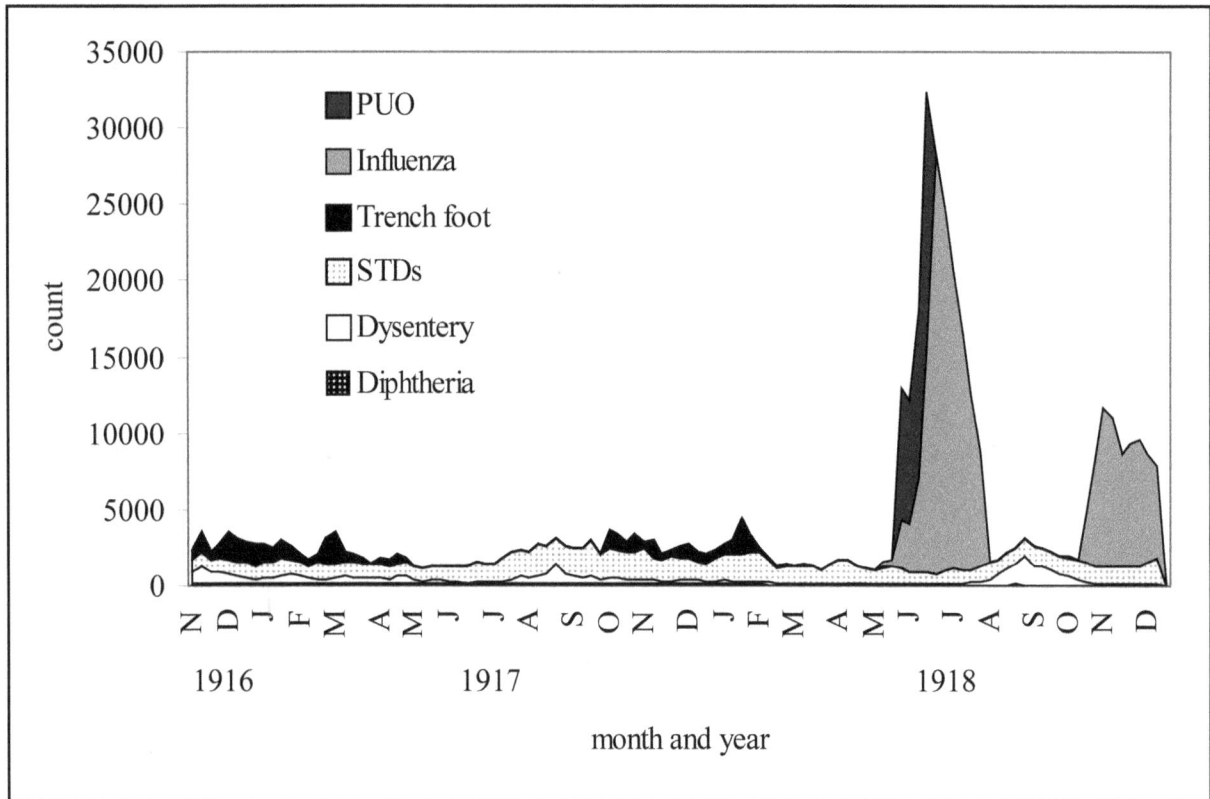

Figure 1. Leading causes of morbidity among British Expeditionary Forces according to the British War Diaries, November 1916 to December 1918.

in the English language since 1743 and that the disease had been endemic in Europe since 1889 (Thompson, 1852; Hall, 1928). In 1918, however, the aetiology of influenza was poorly understood. Viruses were neither filterable nor visible through microscopy. Initially, it was believed that *Bacillus influenzae* was responsible for the outbreak, but sputum studies failed to support this idea (Jordan, 1927). No one knew what was causing otherwise healthy people to sicken and die.

When the first cases of the disease appeared among soldiers in 1918, there was considerable concern about its cause. The BEF had been caught unprepared for chemical warfare in 1915 and was suspicious about agents of biological warfare. When this sudden, if mild, disease hit portions of the Second Army in April of 1918, it was initially labelled as 'PUO', pyrexia of unknown origin. The disease was eventually recognised as a mild form of influenza in mid-May (Soltau, 1918). Influenza was diagnosed by the presence of a suite of symptoms: high fever that lasted for several days, body aches, muscle and joint pain, headache, sore throat, sometimes leading to haemorrhage of the nasal mucous membranes, and cough that sometimes produced a thin, rusty sputum.

In our study, cases of PUO have been categorized with influenza. This may seem unwise, given that the PUO category contained illnesses unrelated to influenza, such as trench fever; furthermore, the volume of official medical statistics for the Great War (Mitchell and Smith, 1931) treats PUO as a category separate from the rest. On

the other hand, the official discussion of the 1918 influenza epidemic on the Western Front conflates influenza and PUO, "The complete figures for the year [for influenza] are not available, but from 18th May to 10th August there were 226,615 admissions, *including pyrexia of uncertain origin*" (emphasis ours) (Mitchell and Smith, 1931: 167). As illustrated in Figure 1, diagnoses of PUO and influenza behaved in a similar manner during the first wave of the 1918 pandemic.

Infectious disease morbidity in the British War Diaries

Figure 1 shows the number of cases (morbidity), by month, of the leading infectious diseases that affected the British Expeditionary Forces in France from November 1916 to December 1918 contained in the British War Diaries. The graph should be read from left to right. Some averaging has been applied because of missing data for sporadic weeks. Note that there are two waves of influenza, shown on the right. The first wave leaps out in June and July of 1918 and the second in October. This is reassuring, for it confirms that the British War Diary data generate the well-documented temporal pattern of influenza morbidity for the summer and autumn outbreaks. Military officials were cautious about discussing the large numbers of sick men during the first wave in the spring and summer, but even if influenza were under-reported, its impact is obvious. It dominates the graph. Another instructive feature of the graph is the close relationship between the two lines that represent

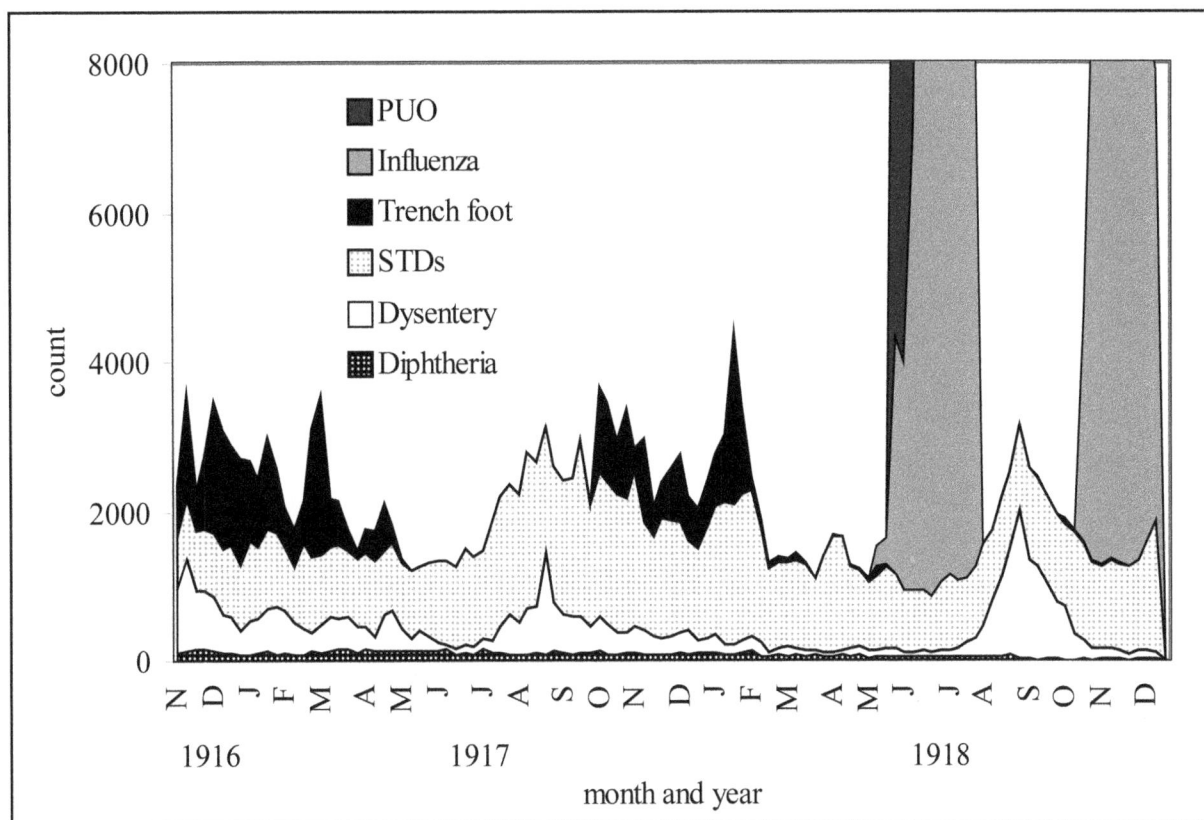

Figure 2. Enlarged scale, Figure 1. Leading causes of morbidity among British Expeditionary Forces according to the British War Diaries, November 1916 to December 1918.

diagnosed cases of PUO and influenza during June and July of 1918. As influenza cases rise in June, so do cases of PUO. By the time of the second wave of influenza in the autumn of 1918, cases of PUO are barely discernible, probably because influenza was made a notifiable disease on the Western Front on 5 October 1918.

An enlarged scale for the graph (Fig. 2) shows the misery that was the lot of soldiers in France during World War I. Sexually transmitted diseases (STDs) — mostly gonorrhoea and syphilis (c.f.: Mitchell and Smith, 1931: 285-86) were a constant problem and figure prominently in the morbidity profile. Standing for days on end in wet, cold, and muddy trenches gave rise to outbreaks of trench foot, which literally caused the feet to rot away, especially in winter. Dysentery and diarrhoea were endemic and peaked during the hot summer months.

But where is influenza in 1916 and 1917? The War Diaries mention sporadic, limited outbreaks among the BEF in France. In December 1916, high rates of influenza were reported among Australian and New Zealand forces (BEF HQ 1916). In May 1917, influenza broke out among dockworkers in Calais, a port about 25 km north of Étaples (BEF HQ 1917). In January 1918, influenza was reported in the port of Marseille in southern France (Gordon, 1918). In the official medical statistics for 1916 to 1920, influenza ranks second to diseases of the digestive system (11.35 and 13.38 percent of all admissions, respectively) as a cause of admission to hospital for soldiers at the Western Front (Mitchell and

Smith, 1931: 286). Although a substantial proportion of this rate comes from the 1918 pandemic, there were 18,894 hospital admissions for influenza in 1916 and 9287 in 1917 (Mitchell and Smith, 1931: 298).

In the BWD data, however, influenza barely shows up in Figures 1 and 2, contrary to what would be expected if a new strain of Influenza A were present. This is not because Medical services personnel were poor diagnosticians: they were trained to recognise unusual forms of respiratory disease. For instance, on January 12 of 1918, Majors Lomer and Hardisty "…proceeded to no 6 Field Ambulance and attended a lecture there on Purulent Bronchitis by Capt Hollis of No 7 Canadian General Hospital." (Canadian War Diaries, 1915-19). Epidemic influenza only emerges as a major disease in the British War Diaries during the late spring of 1918, not before. It was a minor problem of little significance compared to STDs, gastrointestinal infections, trench foot and to the death and destruction associated with the war.

To understand why the profile of morbidity presented by the BWD data would deviate from that derived from hospital admissions, it is necessary to recognize that the sites of observation were different. Soldiers admitted to hospital for treatment for influenza were not representative of all soldiers on the Western Front who suffered from the illness: only the most severe cases would have been evacuated and hospitalized. In effect, the admissions data suffer from hospital patient bias, or Berkson's bias (Berkson, 1946). The BWD data, on the other hand, represent the full spectrum of illnesses, minor and severe, recorded among the troops. From the perspective of soldiers on the ground, and the medical personnel treating them, the BWD data suggest that influenza was a minor problem relative to other common ailments.

Other observations on influenza

The British War Diary entries confirm that a mild form of influenza affected the British Expeditionary Forces from February to June 1918. The BWD entries also indicate that the disease spread from south to north, appearing among BEF troops in Italy in February 1918, but not in northern France until April. The south-to-north spatial pattern raises questions about the 'Étaples-to-everywhere-else' hypothesis.

Diary entries also indicate that soldiers who contracted influenza during the first, mild wave of influenza were not protected from the second, lethal wave. Soldiers ill with influenza in the summer were felled again by the deadly strain circulating in the autumn of 1918 (Newland, 1918). The virulent autumn pandemic seems to have emerged suddenly and the strain seems to have differed from the spring wave. The official medical history of the U.S.A. in WWI also suggests that two different viruses were circulating, based on a north/south divide of the country (Hall, 1928). Edwin Jordan (1927) reached a similar conclusion in 1927 after reviewing these and other pre-1918 outbreaks. This raises a perplexing question: if a severe new strain of Influenza A were already pre-seeded among British forces in Europe, why wasn't the first wave of influenza a virulent one? Moreover, if the virulent form evolved as a result of "small, step-wise mutational changes throughout the viral genome" (Oxford *et al,.* 2002: 113), wouldn't some resistance have been conferred to twice-ill soldiers because of similarities between the ancestral and descendent viruses?

Furthermore, we are unaware of a documentary chain of evidence that shows that military personnel travelling from Europe to the USA prior to the 1918 outbreak either fell sick with influenza (caught in Europe), transmitted it in the USA, or were directly connected to influenza outbreaks on the other side of the Atlantic, such as the herald waves observed in New York City (Olson *et al,.* 2005). In fact, one opinion suggests that influenza appeared "in both Europe and America so nearly at the same time as to render its transference from one area to the other very unlikely" (Hall, 1928: 133).

Conclusions

The perspective on influenza gained from scrutinizing the everyday details of morbidity depicted in the British War Diaries — which cover all illnesses, not just those requiring hospitalization – differs from the picture gained from the official record (Michell and Smith, 1931). Prior to June through August 1918, influenza was a minor illness compared to diarrhoea, dysentery, sexually transmitted diseases, trench foot, and war-related injuries. Influenza/PUO moved from BEF troops in the south, northward to Étaples, not from it. Soldiers who were sick with influenza during the mild, first wave lacked immunity to the virulent, autumn outbreak and fell sick again.

Taken together, the War Diary evidence suggests that the virus associated with the autumn outbreak was new and not pre-seeded among BEF troops years before. Until the genome of the strain associated with the mild wave of influenza from the spring of 1918 is discovered and sequenced, then compared to the genome of the fall strain, this issue will remain unresolved.

That said, Taubenberger and colleagues (2006: E10) recognize that "phylogenetic analysis on its own cannot definitively resolve this issue" [when the lethal virus entered human populations]." In fact, surprising as it may seem, the 1918 pandemic is grossly understudied from a historical, documentary perspective (Phillips, 2004). The documentary evidence is copious but understudied. The biological evidence is sparse: the 1918 influenza pandemic left no imprint on bone but in a few rare instances its viral RNA was preserved. Each type of evidence nevertheless makes it possible to pose questions that can be pursued through the other source (c.f.: Herring and Swedlund, 2003). Together, they offer a richer though still equivocal understanding of the problem. This underlines the importance of using multiple lines of evidence to study disease in the past, a luxury often not afforded to bioarchaeologists who often must work without the benefit of documents.

Acknowledgments

We wish to thank Megan Brickley and Martin Smith for the invitation to present this paper in the Written in Bone session of the 8th Annual Conference for the British Association for Biological Anthropology and Osteoarchaeology at the University of Birmingham. The Wellcome Trust is gratefully acknowledged for funding Herring's travel to present the paper on which this article is based. The paper was improved immeasurably by suggestions from F.G.A. Noon and C. Roberts. This research was funded by a Social Sciences and Humanities Postdoctoral Fellowship (76-2004-0134) and by the Arts Research Board at McMaster University (5-58564). We are grateful to Melissa Stoops and Shobita Ravindran for assistance with data-entry.

Literature cited

Abrahams, A., Hallows, N. and French, H. 1919. "A further investigation into influenza pneumococcal and influenza-streptococcal septica of highly fatal type and its relation to purulent bronchitis." *Lancet* 1: 1-19.

Barry, J.M. 2004a. *The Great Influenza: the Epic Story of the Deadliest Plague in History.* New York: Viking.

Barry, J.M. 2004b. "The site of origin of the 1918 influenza pandemic and its public health implications." *Journal of Translational Medicine* 2: 3.

BEF HQ 1916 British Expeditionary Forces France and Flanders General Headquarters Medical Services, NAUK WO 19 45.

BEF HQ 1917. British Expeditionary Forces France and Flanders General Headquarters Medical Services, NAUK WO 19 46.

BEF HQ 1918. British Expeditionary Forces France and Flanders General Headquarters Medical Services, NAUK WO 19 47.

Berkson, J. 1946. "Limitations of the application of fourfold table analysis to hospital data" *Biometrics Bulletin* 2: 47-53.

Burnet, F.M. and Clark, E. 1942. *Influenza*. London: Macmillan.

Canadian War Diaries 1915-19. Second Canadian Division, NAUK WO 95 4198.

Crosby, A.W. 1989. *America's Forgotten Pandemic: The Influenza of 1918*. Cambridge: Cambridge University Press.

Gordon, P.C.M. 1918. "Memo from the Medical Officer in charge of the Fijian Labour Company to the Assistant Director Medical Services, Marseilles". NAUK WO 95 47.

Hall, M.W. 1928. Chapter II, "Inflammatory Diseases of the Respiratory Tract (bronchitis; influenza; bronchopneumonia; lobar pneumonia)," in Siler, J.F. (ed.), *Communicable Diseases, The Medical Department of the United States Army in the World War* Vol. IX, 61-169.

Hammond, J.A.R., Rolland, W. and Shore T.H.G. 1917. "Purulent bronchitis: a study of cases occurring amongst the British troops at a base in France." *Lancet* 2: 41-5.

Herring, D.A. and Swedlund, A.C. (eds.) 2003. *Human Biologists in the Archives*. Cambridge: Cambridge University Press.

Jordan, E.O. 1927. *Epidemic Influenza. A Survey*. Chicago: American Medical Association.

Kobasa, D., Jones, S.M., Shinya, K., Kash, J. C., Copps, J., Ebihafra, H., Hattsa, Y, Kim, J.H., Halfmann, P., Hatta, M., Feldmann, F., Alimonti, J.B., Fernando, L., Li, Y., Katze, M.G., Feldmann, H. and Kawaoka, Y. 2007. Aberrant innate immune response in lethal infection of macaques with the 1918 influenza virus. *Nature* 445: 319-323.

Mitchell, Maj. T.J. and Smith, G.M. 1931. *History of the Great War Based on Official Documents. Medical Services. Casualties and Medical Statistics of the Great War*. London: HMSO.

NAUK refers to files of the National Archives of the UK.

Newland, F.R. 1918. "Notes on the Incidence and Dissemination of Malaria in Italy with a statistical table and two explanatory maps". NAUK WO 95 4198.

Olson, D.R., Simonsen, L., Edelson, P.J. and Morse, S.S. 2005. "Epidemiological evidence of an early wave of the 1918 influenza pandemic in New York City." *Proceedings of the National Academy of Science U.S.A.* 102: 11059-63.

Oxford, J.S., Sefton, A., Jackson, R., Innes, W., Daniels, R.S. and Johnson, N.P. 2002. "World War I may have allowed the emergence of "Spanish" influenza." *Lancet Infectious Disease* 2: 111-4.

Oxford, J. S., Lambkin, R., Sefton, A., Daniels, R., Elliot, A., Brown, R. and Gill, D. 2005. "A hypothesis: the conjunction of soldiers, gas, pigs, ducks, geese and horses in Northern France during the Great War provided the conditions for the emergence of the "Spanish" influenza pandemic of 1918-1919." *Vaccine* 23: 940-945.

Patterson, K.D. and Pyle, G.F. 1991. "The geography and mortality of the 1918 influenza pandemic." *Bulletin of the History of Medicine* 65: 4-21.

Phillips, H. 2004. "The re-appearing shadow of 1918: trends in the historiography of the 1918-19 influenza pandemic." *Canadian Bulletin of Medical History* 21: 121-134.

Reid, A.H., Fanning, T.G., Hultin, J.V. and Taubenberger, J.K. 1999. "Origin and evolution of the 1918 "Spanish" influenza virus hemagglutinin gene." *Proceedings of the National Academy of Science* 96: 1651-6.

Scholtissek, C. 1992. "Cultivating a killer virus." *Natural History* 1: 3-6.

Scholtissek, C. 1994. "Source for influenza pandemics." *European Journal of Epidemiology* 4: 455-458.

Soltau, B. 1918. "Note on a Mild Pyrexial Epidemic, Resembling Influenza, May 12, 1918". NAUK WO 95 47.

Taubenberger, J.K., Reid, A.H., Lourens, R.M., Wang, R., Jin, G. and Fanning, T.G. 2005. "Characterization of the 1918 influenza virus polymerase genes." *Nature* 437: 889-93.

Taubenberger, J.K. and Morens, D.M. 2006. "1918 influenza: the mother of all pandemics." *Emerging Infectious Diseases* 12: 15-22.

Taubenberger, J.K., Reid, A.H., Lourens, R.M., Wang, R., Jin, G. and Fanning, T.G. 2006. "Taubenberger *et al.* reply." *Nature* 440: E9-10.

Thompson, T. 1852. *Annals of Influenza or Epidemic Cattarhal fever in Great Britain from 1510 to 1837.* London: The Sydenham Society.

U.S. Surgeon General. 1919. *Annual Report of the Surgeon General for Fiscal Year 1919, Volume I, Infectious Diseases.* Washington.

Combining palaeopathological and historical evidence for health in the Crusades

Piers D. Mitchell

Imperial College London, 84 Huntingdon Road, London, N2 9DU
e-mail address for correspondence: piers.mitchell@imperial.ac.uk

Abstract

In most countries training in history and physical anthropology/osteoarchaeology has traditionally been separate. In this paper I hope to illustrate the advantages of combining evidence from both approaches. A number of biological anthropologists are using this combined approach already and I certainly do not claim to be the first. Here I will consider some of the ways in which I have found it helpful in my understanding of the medical history of the crusades.

In this overview there are examples of the interplay between the texts written by crusaders in the twelfth and thirteenth centuries and excavated human skeletal remains and human intestinal parasite ova from the time of the crusades. The sites discussed are the city of Caesarea, the city of Acre, the village of Parvum Gerinum, and the castles of Vadum Iacob and Vallis Moysis. Here all of these sites are considered in order to discuss the archaeological and historical evidence for the possible removal of arrows by battlefield orderlies, manipulation and splinting of tibial fractures by surgeons, the interaction between hygiene and parasitic worms, and life expectancy for different populations.

Using written as well as archaeological sources to address challenging hypotheses has considerable advantages when investigating health in the past. We should also encourage those who wish to train in both fields.

Keywords: written texts; student training; health; crusades; palaeopathology

Introduction

Most of us in the fields of biological anthropology and osteoarchaeology undertake our research from a fundamentally archaeological perspective. The core principal behind the study of these areas is the analysis of skeletal material from the past that has been excavated from the ground. Training in these disciplines focuses on how to obtain material for analysis from a reliable archaeological context, followed by laboratory-based research to maximize the information we can acquire from such material. Those researching time periods before humans invented written or pictorial methods of communication have little option but to concentrate solely on the archaeological approach. However, the vast majority of excavated human skeletal material comes from time periods when those communities had developed the ability to write. In consequence, a huge amount of information concerning the anthropology of these past populations can be obtained from reading their records.

Some biological anthropologists have undergone further specialist training in areas that require particular knowledge and experience in order to perform reliably and accurately. Such areas include bone and dental isotopes, ancient DNA, histology, forensic facial reconstruction, and the use of ancient written texts. It is these texts written in languages that are no longer used in modern populations that I will discuss here. I am not trained in aDNA or isotopes, for example, so have worked with colleagues in collaborations in my research. This is what most biological anthropologists do when they need information from ancient textual sources, and

they approach a historian. In some circumstances this has worked very well, with the Battle of Towton excavation being one good example (Fiorato *et al.*, 2000). Unfortunately, this is not always easy as historians are not necessarily interested in the same questions as anthropologists. To use an example in my own field of interest, palaeopathologists generally want to know what diseases were present in a population, while medical historians generally want to know how people in that population perceived their illness and how ill health affected the social community. Many medical historians avoid attempting retrospective diagnosis, as such information is often not relevant to their research goals. In contrast, retrospective diagnosis is central to the goals of palaeopathologists. This apparent incompatibility between palaeopathologists and medical historians is perhaps one reason why there has been only limited integration of research in these superficially similar fields.

I believe that the most reliable way for biological anthropologists to obtain information from the written sources, that is relevant to the past populations they study, is to read the texts themselves. In this way they can search out the specific information relevant to their needs. To do this they would need to be trained not only in the language of that population, but also in how to interpret texts written from the unique perspective of that past community. It is important that quotes from past authors are not merely taken at face value, but that modern interpretation includes knowledge of who the author was, their reason for writing, the literary style with which they chose to write, the readership audience, their biases and attitudes, and their sources of information. Ideally the text should be read in the language in which it was written, to reduce the risk misinterpretation due to a suboptimal or out of date translation by others. Such an approach is not as difficult as we might first think, especially where English language translations have been published to act as a starting point for students to use in parallel with these original texts. It has been used with success at undergraduate level, for example on the course on Disease in the Past by the History of Medicine Unit at Imperial College London School of Medicine.

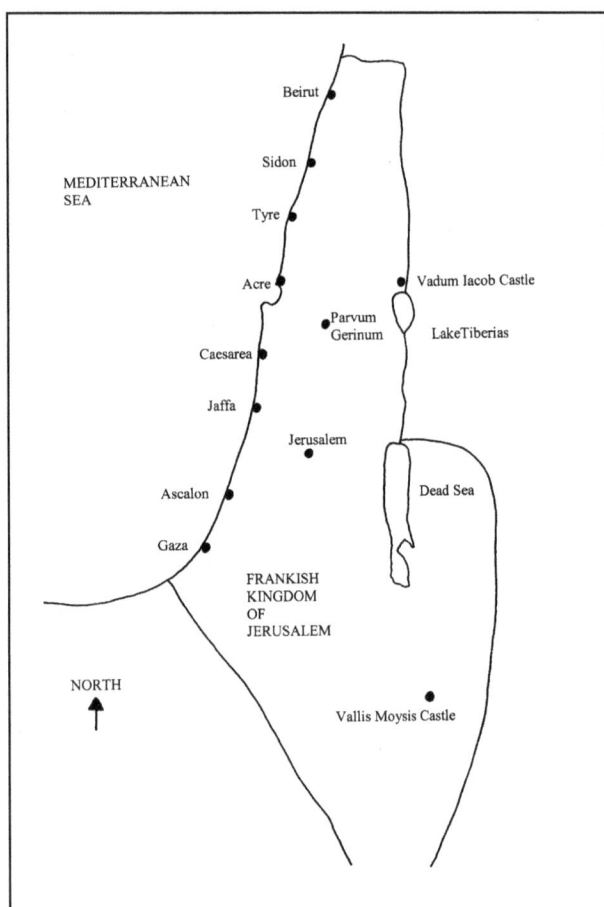

Figure 1. Map of the Frankish Kingdom of Jerusalem, with borders as of the mid-twelfth century.

In this paper I discuss some examples where information from written sources has enabled me to interpret bioarchaeological contexts better than would otherwise have been the case if such written sources were unavailable to me. My aim is not to give examples of textual and bioarchaeological integration in widely different geographical areas and different time periods, but rather to concentrate on just the one example of the medieval Middle East. Nor do I intend this to be a proof of the superiority of one technique over another, but rather an illustration of how an individual can combine information from both approaches in an attempt to gain a more robust interpretation of life in the past. This would not have been possible simply by collaborating with historians, as the medical history community had not shown any interest in health or disease in the sites I was excavating. A consequence of this lack of interest was

that virtually all the textual information would have been unavailable to biological anthropologists had the original source texts not been consulted. The majority of the sources were written in medieval Latin or French, but some were in Arabic, Syriac, or Greek. This is not the place for an in depth critique of the range of written texts mentioning disease and medicine that date from the crusades, but such a discussion is available elsewhere (Mitchell 2004b). The sites discussed are marked on a map of the region, to highlight their geographic relationship with one another and with the borders of the Frankish Kingdom of Jerusalem (Fig. 1).

Health on the battlefield

The castle of Jacob's Ford (Vadum Iacob) was the site of a great battle in Galilee in 1179AD (Ibn Shaddad, 2001; Ellenblum, 2003). Around a thousand troops of the crusader king of Jerusalem and the Knights Templar were besieged in the castle by the army of Saladin, the Sultan of Egypt. The outer wall of the castle and one vaulted internal building had been completed, but the rest of the castle was still under construction. The walls were undermined with a tunnel and the castle was stormed. Excavation has found no evidence for the use of the site as military stronghold at any time before or after this one year period (1178-9), and it was raised to the ground and abandoned at the end of the battle. The bodies of a number of the defending soldiers were recovered lying in a layer of ash under a crusader style vaulted building that collapsed in the ensuing fire. These demonstrate a range of blade injuries from sword blows, and arrow-heads found either embedded in the bone or in areas where soft tissues would have been present during life (Mitchell *et al.*, 2006). Used arrows have been found scattered right across the site, some retaining straight tips and others with their points turned over (Fig. 2). Archaeological evidence for these showers of arrows has also been found at other sites in the medieval Middle East (Mitchell, 2004a; Rafael and Tepper, 2005). One might expect that these arrows would retain their sharp points if entering human flesh and only develop a bent tip if they hit as hard surface such as a defensive castle wall. However, publications by surgeons on arrow wounds from nineteenth century north America have shown how iron tips often turned over on impact with the human body (Bill, 1862; Wilson, 1901; Milner, 2005). In consequence the presence of a straight or curved tip cannot be used to differentiate whether an arrow hit an opposing soldier or merely bounced off the castle wall or landed in the soil.

In one corner of this vaulted building in the castle a collection of fifteen arrow-heads was found by the excavators. Since they were underneath the vault they could not have been fired there directly from outside the castle walls. The arrows were scattered on the ground in differing orientations, not closely packed and parallel as might have been the case had they been stored there bound together. Their alignment was parallel to the floor. Those excavating the site thought that a defending soldier might have been cornered here, and that these were the remains of those arrows fired at him by Muslim archers that missed his body. Another possibility is that arrows fired into the castle during the siege were collected up and placed here for a blacksmith to resharpen, and allow their reuse. However, no blacksmith's hearth or tools were found in this room. A further hypothesis worth considering is one suggested by reading crusader accounts of battles such as this. This may perhaps represent evidence for battlefield medical treatment.

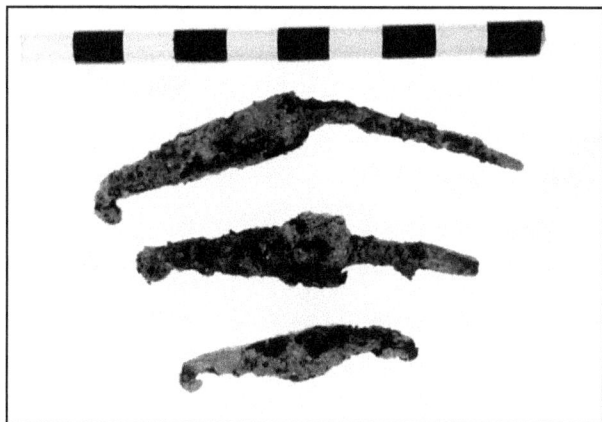

Figure 2. Three of the thousands of arrowheads recovered from the battle of Vadum Iacob castle, 1179AD. Reproduced with permission from Mitchell, P.D. *Medicine in the Crusades: Warfare, Wounds and the Medieval Surgeon*. Cambridge University Press 2004.

A number of crusader soldiers wrote down their experiences during battles in which they took part (Ambroise, 1897; John of Joinville 1874; Minstrel of Reims, 1876). They often mention how each army would shower the other with arrows before horsemen charged with lances and swords. Crusader soldiers usually wore armour that helped protect them from arrows. These included an outer coat of chain mail, and a thick padded jerkin beneath this called a *gambeson* (Nicolle, 1988; Edge and Paddock, 1996). Those arrows that penetrated the rings of the mail were often stopped by the dense, padded layer below. Only the arrows that passed through both these layers actually caused injuries.

A number of crusader writings mention that soldiers removed these arrows in the battlefield, while the difficult cases required extraction by a surgeon accompanying the army (Mitchell, 2004b). Texts from the 1180s (the time of this battle) mentioned how four surgeons from the Order of St. John accompanied the crusader army into battle, and treated the wounded in tents (Kedar, 1998).

Medical texts from Europe that were written at the time of the crusades give details as to how such arrows could be removed (Theodorich Borgognoni, 1498:112v; Paterson, 1988). If they could not be pulled out the way they went in, there were several options. A medical instrument could be slid down the shaft of the arrow to cover the barbs, and so allow its extraction without the barbs catching on the soft tissues. Alternatively, the arrow could be pushed right through the body until it

came out the other side. Finally, the arrow could be left where it was for a few days while the soft tissues around it decomposed, so the arrow could be pulled out more easily.

One possibility is that the collection of arrowheads in the corner of this building may represent a pile of arrows extracted from wounded soldiers during this battle. It would have been logical that the wounded would have been treated in the only building within the castle to have a completed roof, to protect the injured from arrows fired over the walls. A surgeon might have had his table at this end of the building, and tossed the arrows he extracted into the corner of the room. This is a procedure that the manuscript sources confirm did occur on a regular basis, but is very difficult to identify in an archaeological context. While we may never know for sure which of the explanations is the correct one, it is a possibility that the pile of arrowheads is all that remains of a battlefield treatment centre.

Health in towns and cities

Excavation of crusader towns and cities comes with its own challenges, but has great potential to tell us huge amounts if we are able to interpret its complexity. In contrast to the undifferentiated bodies on a battlefield, or the single cemeteries that exist at most smaller communities such as villages, cities give us a number of distinct cemeteries. If we can understand how a population decided to bury different people in different places, then life expectancy, health, burial practices and a host of other factors can be compared between the different social groups. We can also compare the life experience of people who chose to live in cities with those who lived elsewhere.

Trauma can be a good way to compare different lifestyles, as different occupations may cause injuries to different parts of the body. Furthermore, fractures in adults often leave permanent changes to the skeleton. As mentioned earlier, there were many battles and skirmishes that took place during the crusades, and so we would expect people exposed to warfare to have either fresh or healed weapon injuries on their skeletal remains. In contrast, communities protected from warfare but still exposed to workplace accidents and bar brawls would tend to show a different pattern of fractures. The cemeteries of the port city of Caesarea Maritima have been analyzed for evidence of trauma (Mitchell, 2006a), and the findings compared with that of the garrison of Jacob's Ford castle, known to have died a violent death in warfare (Mitchell *et al.*, 2006). It was expected that the population of Caesarea would show a mixture of both industrial accidents and interpersonal weaponless violence on the one hand, and weapon injuries from participation in warfare on the other. However, in over 150 skeletons, no evidence for weapon injuries from the crusader period population of Caesarea has been found so far (Smith and Zegerson, 1999; Mitchell, 2006a). This is despite the presence of a mandible fracture (Fig.3), compatible with a fist fight (Krenkel, 1994), three examples of vertebral fractures, seven tibia and femur fractures all compatible with falls, and a depressed skull fracture compatible with either a fall onto the head or a heavy object landing on the head. All of these fractures were well healed and remodeled, none being perimortem. This pattern suggests the crusader population at Caesarea maintained a peaceful lifestyle punctuated by intermitted industrial accidents and drunken bar brawls, rather than a military lifestyle.

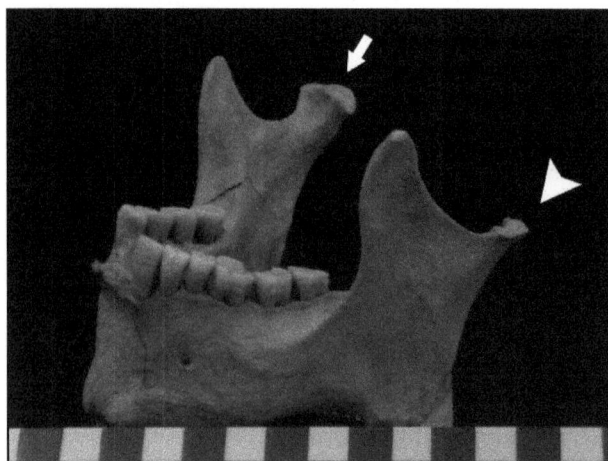

Figure 3. Mandible fracture from Caesarea, 12-13th century AD. Small arrow shows normal right mandibular condyle, and broad arrow highlights fracture nonunion at mandibular neck on the left side. Reproduced with permission from Mitchell, P.D. *Medicine in the Crusades: Warfare, Wounds and the Medieval Surgeon.* Cambridge University Press 2004.

This was not at all what was expected, so the written sources from crusader times were then consulted to see what evidence there was for lifestyle in the port cities of the Mediterranean coast. It seems that Caesarea contained sailors from the ships that transported pilgrims and crusaders to and from Europe. There were inns and accommodation for the pilgrims, as well as guides to take them to the holy places. There were merchants to import and export goods, as the ports acted as western termini of the silk route to the east. It also contained clergy to service the cathedral, churches and monasteries of the city. Caesarea had robust defensive walls but was not a major military centre (Holum *et al.*, 1988; Raban and Holum, 1996). The historical sources explain the pattern of trauma noted in the skeletal remains. There seems to have been little exposure to warfare but plenty of exposure to those industrial accidents to which sailors, craftsmen, builders, publicans and similar manual occupations are prone. Written sources were also illuminating regarding the standard of medical practice expected of surgeons treating such fractures in the kingdom of Jerusalem. Medical negligence legislation dating from the first half of the thirteenth century stated that if a doctor treated a patient with a broken leg, but applied useless plasters so the bone healed at an angle and the patient became disabled, the doctor was guilty of negligence. If the patient were a slave, the doctor would

be obliged to buy the slave from his owner. However, if he crippled a free man, the surgeon would have his right thumb cut off (Kausler, 1839). This would have prevented him from practicing medicine ever again, as he would have been unable to hold surgical instruments. This might explain why the long bone fractures discovered so far at Caesarea appear to have healed in reasonably good alignment, as the surgeons would have been under considerable pressure to treat such fractures well (Mitchell, 2006a).

Another aspect of life for which medieval cities were well renowned was the smell from human and animal waste left out in the streets. To investigate this topic further, the latrines, cesspools and drains of another crusader port city, that of Acre, have been the subject of an ongoing interdisciplinary study (Mitchell and Tepper, 2007; Syon *et al.*, in press). One of the aims is to understand gastrointestinal parasites in the crusader population. The largest latrine so far analysed was that in the complex of the Order of St. John (Mitchell and Stern, 2001). This thirteenth century latrine was comprised of thirty-five toilet seats, was built on four floors, and water collected from the roof was used to flush the excrement down into the basement. It fell into disuse once the crusaders left Acre in 1291. Samples were analyzed from those areas of the basement latrine soil that were radiocarbon dated to the thirteenth century. A further crusader period cesspool from Acre has also been analyzed (Mitchell and Tepper, in press). This was built in the floor of a complex of crusader buildings dating from the thirteenth century. The cesspool was built in the crusader masonry style, in the floor of a crusader building. A number of crusader coins were recovered from the contents, and no coins were found dating from the Islamic periods before or after the crusades. These factors suggest that its use was limited to the crusader period. The human faecal waste in this latrine and cesspool included the eggs of many parasitic worms from the intestines of those using the facilities. The most commonly found was the whipworm, *Trichuris trichuria* (Fig. 4). The next most common was the roundworm, *Ascaris lumbricoides*. Also found were the pork/beef tapeworm (*Taenia sp.*) and the fish tapeworm (*Diphyllobothrium latum*). The fish tapeworm has never before been identified in the Middle East, but was common in northern Europe during the medieval period (Mitchell and Stern, 2001). This suggests that it may have been deposited in these latrines by crusaders from northern Europe (Mitchell *et al.*, in press).

Historical texts were consulted to understand attitudes to hygiene in crusader cities, and to determine what the medical profession thought of these parasitic worms. It seems that the port cities of the Frankish states in the Latin East were very dirty places, even by medieval standards. When the Muslim traveler Ibn Jubayr visited Acre in 1184, he wrote that, 'it stinks and is filthy, being full of refuse and excrement' (Ibn Jubayr, 1952: 318). This was the only city where he made a point of mentioning the smell in his travels around the entire Mediterranean, so this was not just his way of suggesting the Christians were less hygienic than Muslim cities. It seems Acre was particularly bad. The fact that someone built this latrine and cesspool shows that all human waste was not just dumped onto the streets, but it does seem that enough was dumped there to cause quite a stench. Medical texts of the time also mention these worms. Maurus of Salerno was head master of this famous medieval medical centre of learning in Italy in the 1170s-1190s. He wrote of the various forms of intestinal parasitic worms known at that time in his work The Commentary on the Prognostics of Hippocrates (Saffron, 1972). He described intestinal worms as long or short and as flat or round. Comparison with modern parasitological texts (Muller and Baker, 1990) suggest that the long round ones were probably Ascaris, the short round ones probably Trichuris, the short flat ones probably single tapeworm segments and the long flat ones probably several tapeworm segments still attached together. These worms were not in themselves thought worthy of treatment by medieval doctors, as they were not perceived as a parasite or disease. Rather, Maurus and his peers believed the worms to have been created by an excess of phlegm in the body, phlegm being one of the four humours. The passing of worms with the stool was a sign of a phlegmatic state, and it was this, not the worms themselves, that medieval doctors tried to treat with dietary modification and bloodletting.

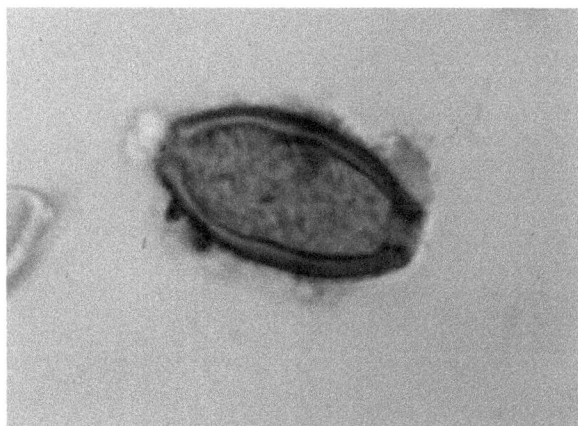

Figure 4: Whipworm ovum from a cesspool in Acre, dating from the 13th century AD.

Health variation between sites

This approach can be used in reverse, of course. Rather than using textual sources to help explain archaeological finds, questions raised by written sources can be answered using archaeological excavations. The comparison of two contrasting sites is a common and sensible approach in physical anthropology. In some cases it is the archaeological findings that are used to draw conclusions as to whether the populations will be contrasting or not, and so trigger the anthropological comparison. However, textual sources can also be helpful in this regard. Written sources from the crusader period show how poorly defended rural settlements were easily looted and burned by raiding parties from across the kingdom's borders, but cities and castles were often passed by on account of their strong walls, dry moat, and

defending soldiers (Albert of Aachen, 2007; Ernoul, 1871). This might suggest that the safest place to live would be well-defended sites such as castles or cities. However, written sources also describe how smelly, polluted and overcrowded some fortified settlements were (Ibn Jubayr, 1952: 318). The poor sanitation and overcrowding may have increased the spread of infectious diseases. A range of infectious diseases have been identified as present in the medieval Middle East, and often city dwellers fled to the countryside during an outbreak of an epidemic (Mitchell, 2003; Mitchell, in press). Provisioning may have been different between fortified and rural sites too, as castles would have to buy in food that could be stored, while farming villages could grow their own fresh food. In consequence, the written manuscripts show that health inequalities may well have existed between rural and fortified sites, but do not clearly show which might have been the healthiest places to live.

One archaeological approach to this question has been to compare health at the rural farming village of Parvum Gerinum with the castle of Vallis Moysis (Mitchell, 2006b). Both of these lay in the crusader kingdom of Jerusalem, and were inhabited during the twelfth century. For several reasons the comparison was undertaken using the immature individuals. Firstly the habit of burying children separately from adults in the medieval Middle East means that the children's section was fully excavated in both sites. No adults were buried within the walls of the castle site, and only four adults were excavated intact from the village site by the time the excavation was discontinued. Secondly, the age at death of the developing skeleton can be determined quite accurately compared with adults, using dental eruption, epiphyseal formation and fusion, and long bone length in the fetus (Scheuer and Black, 2000).

The age at death profile for both sites (Figure 5) were of a type we see today in the poorest developing world countries (Murray and Lopez, 1996: 175), again suggesting that the samples were probably representative of the medieval population at each site. It was found that children tended to die at an older age at the farming village (n.=50) than at the castle (n.=15), and the difference was statistically significant on Mann-Whitney U-test (p=0.05). At the castle 60% of child deaths had occurred before they were one month old, while at the farming village it was only by the age of one year that 60% of child deaths had occurred. While a larger sample would clearly have been desirable at the castle, enough individuals were still available for the difference to be highlighted on statistical analysis.

Modern medical studies of developing world populations have shown that children tend to die from different causes at different ages (Murray and Lopez, 1996: table 5.3; Seear, 2000: 7; Moss *et al.*, 2002). Applying these modern findings to the medieval samples suggests interesting contrasts between the two sites. Children who die around the time of birth tend to succumb due to birth trauma or asphyxia from difficult labour, intrauterine

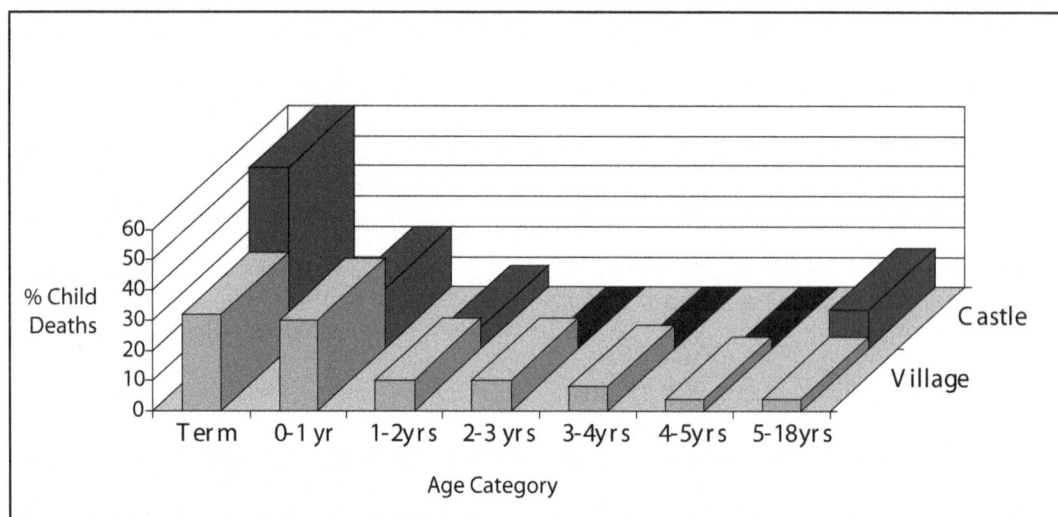

Figure 5. Childhood deaths at the castle of Vallis Moysis and the farming village of Parvum Gerinum (village site n.=50, castle site n.=15).

infections, or congenital malformations. These problems seem to have been common at the castle site. Children that die aged between one month and one year tend to die from infectious diseases such as measles, whooping cough, and tetanus, as well as those who survived a few months with congenital malformations and intrauterine infections. These childhood infectious diseases seem to have been more common causes of death at the village site.

Integrating the written and archaeological evidence for life expectancy at the farming village and castle is very interesting. In times of peace it was probably safest if the medieval population brought up their families in a farming village. However, in times of war it might have been safer to move to a strongly fortified castle or city to protect themselves from raiding parties.

Having considered some of the benefits of complementing bioarchaeological research with textual sources, it is also worth considering whether there may be any negative consequences of not utilizing these sources. In my own experience I feel more at risk of drawing erroneous conclusions regarding population health if I do not have access to complementary textual sources. I am aware that any sampling bias or mistakes in archaeological interpretation may lead me to draw incorrect conclusions. Some form of textual evidence has survived for the vast majority of populations that are studied by biological anthropologists. Over the next generation I hope it will become the norm for a much greater proportion of us to be trained in the skills needed to study life in the past using both techniques. If we do not, then as a profession the accuracy of our conclusions may be much lower than we would hope.

Conclusion

Here I have tried to highlight the value of the balanced use of both historical and anthropological sources in understanding life in the past. If original historical sources had not been consulted, none of the above studies would have taken place in their complete form. Without written descriptions of battlefield medical treatment, the possibility of battlefield treatment locations would not be considered at excavation. In the absence of textual evidence for medical negligence laws, the significance of healed fracture alignment would be missed. The mere existence of parasitic helminth ova in crusader latrines and cesspools would be of only minor importance without written descriptions of hygiene in these cities and the recorded views of medical practitioners of the time regarding these worms. It would not necessarily occur to us to compare life expectancy at a crusader castle and a village if the texts had not suggested potential health inequalities between the two lifestyles.

Literature cited

Albert of Aachen. 2007. *Historia Iherosolimitana.* S. Edgington (ed.), Oxford: Oxford Medieval Texts.

Ambroise. 1897. *Estoire de Guerre Sainte: Histoire en Vers de la Troisième Croisade (1190-1192)*. G. Paris (ed.). Paris: Imprimerie Nationale.

Bill, J.H. 1862. "Notes on arrow wounds". *American Journal of the Medical Sciences* 44: 365-87.

Edge, D., and Paddock, J.M. 1996. *Arms and Armor of the Medieval Knight.* London: Saturn Books.

Ellenblum, R. 2003. "Frontier activities: the transformation of a Muslim sacred site into the Frankish castle of Vadum Iacob". *Crusades* 2: 83-97.

Ernoul. 1871. *Chronicle d'Ernoul et de Bernard le Trésorier*. M.L. de Mas Latiré (ed.). Paris: Jules Renouard.

Fiorato, V., Boylston, A., and Knusel, C. (eds.) 2000. *Blood Red Roses. The Archaeology of a Mass Grave from the Battle of Towton, AD 1461*. Oxford: Oxbow.

Holum, K.G., Hohlfelder, R.L., Bull, R.J., and Raban, A. 1988. *King Herod's Dream: Caesarea on the Sea*. New York: W.W. Norton.

Ibn Jubayr. 1952. *The Travels of Ibn Jubayr*. (ed. & trans.) Broadhurst, R.C.J.. London: Jonathan Cape.

Ibn Shaddad. 2001. *The Rare and Excellent History of Saladin*. (ed. & trans.) Richards, D.S. Aldershot: Ashgate.

John of Joinville. 1874. *Histoire de Saint Louis. Jean Sire de Joinville*. (ed.) de Wailly. N. Paris: Librairie de Firmin Didot Frères.

Kausler, E.H. (ed.). 1839. *Assises de Jerusalem. Les Livres des Assises et des Usages de Reaume de Jerusalem*. Stuttgart: Adolf Krabbe, document 231.

Kedar, B.Z. 1998. A twelfth century description of the Jerusalem Hospital. In: Nicholson, H. (ed.) *The Military Orders. Volume 2. Welfare and Warfare*. Aldershot: Ashgate. 3-26.

Krenkel, C. (1994) *Biomechanics and Osteosynthesis of Condylar Neck Fractures of the Mandible*. Chicago: Quintessence.

Milner G.R. 2005. "Nineteenth-century arrow wounds and perceptions of prehistoric warfare" *American Antiquity* 70: 144-56.

Minstrel of Reims. 1876. *Récits d'un Ménestrel de Reims au Treizième Siècle*. (ed.) de Wailly, N. Paris: Librairie de la Société de l'Histoire de France.

Mitchell, P.D. 2003. "Pre-Columbian treponemal disease from 14th century AD Safed, Israel and the implications for the medieval eastern Mediterranean" *American Journal of Physical Anthropology* 121: 117-24.

Mitchell, P.D. 2004a. "The palaeopathology of skulls recovered from a medieval cave cemetery at Safed, Israel (thirteenth to seventeenth century)" *Levant* 36: 243-50.

Mitchell, P.D. 2004b. *Medicine in the Crusades: Warfare, Wounds and the Medieval Surgeon*. Cambridge: Cambridge University Press.

Mitchell, P.D. 2006a. "Trauma in the crusader period city of Caesarea: a major port in the medieval eastern Mediterranean" *International Journal of Osteoarchaeology* 16: 493-505.

Mitchell, P.D. 2006b. "Child health in the crusader period inhabitants of Tel Jezreel, Israel" *Levant* 38: 37-44.

Mitchell, P.D. (in press) "The spread of disease with the crusades". In: Nance, B. and Glaze, E.F. (eds.) *Between Text and Patient: The Medical Enterprise in Medieval and Early Modern Europe*. Florence: Sismel.

Mitchell, P.D., Nagar, Y. and Ellenblum, R. 2006. "Weapon injuries in the 12th century crusader garrison of Vadum Iacob castle, Galilee" *International Journal of Osteoarchaeology* 16: 145-55.

Mitchell, P.D., Huntley, J., and Sterns, E. (in press) "Bioarchaeological analysis of the 13th century latrines of the crusader hospital of St. John at Acre, Israel". In: Zajac, W. (ed.) *The Military Orders: volume 3. Their History and Heritage*. Aldershot: Ashgate.

Mitchell, P.D. and Stern, E. 2001. "Parasitic intestinal helminth ova from the latrines of the 13th century crusader hospital of St. John in Acre, Israel". In: La Verghetta, M., and Capasso, L. (eds.) *Proceedings of the XIIIth European Meeting of the Palaeopathology Association, Chieti Italy*. Teramo: Edigrafital S.p.A. 207-13.

Mitchell, P.D. and Tepper, Y. (2007) "Intestinal parasitic worm eggs from a crusader period cesspool in the city of Acre (Israel)". *Levant* 39: 91-95.

Moss W., Darmstadt G.L, Marsh, D.R., Black R.E., and Santosham, M. 2002. "Research priorities for the reduction of perinatal and neonatal morbidity and mortality in developing country communities". *Journal of Perinatology* 22: 484-95.

Muller, R. and Baker, J.R. 1990. *Medical Parasitology*. Philadelphia: J.B Lippincott.

Murray, C.J.L., and Lopez, A.D. 1996. *The Global Burden of Disease*. Boston: Harvard School of Public Health.

Nicolle, D. 1988. *Arms and Armour in the Crusading Era, 1050-1350*. 2 vols. New York: Kraus.

Paterson, L.M. 1988. "Military surgery: knights, sergeants and Raimon of Avignon's version of the Chirurgia of Roger of Salerno (1180-1209)". In: Harper-Bill, C. and Harvey, R. (eds.) *The Ideals and Practice of Medieval Knighthood II*. Woodbridge: Boydell Press. 117-46.

Raban, A. and Holum, K.G. 1996. *Caesarea Maritima: a Retrospective After Two Millennia*. Leiden: E.J. Brill.

Rafael, K. and Tepper, Y. 2005. "The archaeological evidence for the Mamluk siege of Arsuf". *Mamluk Studies Review* 9: 85-100.

Riley-Smith, J.S.C. (ed.) 1999. *The Oxford History of the Crusades*. Oxford: Oxford University Press.

Saffron, M.H. 1972. "Maurus of Salerno. A twelfth century "optimus physicus" with his commentary on the

Prognostics of Hippocrates" *Transactions of the American Philosophical Society* 62: 5-104.

Scheuer, L, and Black, S. 2000. *Developmental Juvenile Osteology*. San Diego: Academic Press.

Seear, M.D. 2000. *Manual of Tropical Pediatrics*. Cambridge: Cambridge University Press.

Setton K.M., (ed.) 1955-89. *A History of the Crusades*. 6 vols. Philadelphia: University of Pennsylvania Press (vol.1) and Madison: University of Wisconsin (vols.2-6).

Smith, P, and Zegerson, T. 1999. "Morbidity and mortality in post-Byzantine populations from Caesarea". In: Holum K, Raban A, and Patrich J, (eds.). *Caesarea Papers 2: Herod's Temple, the Provincial Governor's Praetorium and Granaries, the Later Harbor, a Gold Coin Hoard and Other Studies*. Portsmouth (Rhode Island): Journal of Roman Archaeology. 433-40.

Syon, D, Stern, E. and Mitchell, P.D. (in press). "Water installations at Crusader Akko". *'Atiqot*.

Theodorich Borgognoni. 1498. "Cyrurgia". In: Locatellus, B. (ed.) *Cyrurgia Guidonis de Chauliaco, et Cyrurgia Bruni, Theoderici, Rogerii, Rolandi, Bertapali, Lanfranci*. Venice: 106-146.

Wilson, T. 1901. "Arrow wounds" *American Anthropologist* 3: 513-31.

When hard work is disease: the interpretation of enthesopathies

Charlotte Henderson

Department of Archaeology, Durham University, Science Site, South Road, Durham, DH1 3LE
e-mail address for correspondence: c.y.henderson@durham.ac.uk

Abstract

Enthesopathies, lytic lesions or bone spurs at sites of tendon, ligament or joint capsule attachments to bone, can be seen in radiographs, in cadaver samples and human skeletal remains. Many factors can contribute to their formation. However, it is the relationship between appendicular enthesopathies and physical exertion (or repetitive labour) that has captured the imagination of bioarchaeologists. In this context they are called musculoskeletal stress markers (MSM). Whilst there are clinical papers which discuss stress induced enthesopathy formation, they generally focus on disease processes (particularly the seronegative spondyloarthropathies) associated with enthesopathies. There are bioarchaeological papers discussing disease related enthesopathy formation, but compared to that on MSM, the research is negligible.

This study explores the relationship between enthesopathies in the upper limb and bone-forming diseases. Clinical literature was reviewed and a list of diseases known to cause enthesopathy formation in the appendicular skeleton compiled. General diagnostic criteria for these diseases were created and used to divide skeletons from the late medieval site of Fishergate House, York into two groups: 1) disease free; 2) possible enthesopathy forming disease. Chi-square tests (p<0.05) were used to compare the frequencies of upper limb enthesopathies in groups 1 and 2. It was hypothesised that the skeletons with 'diseases' would have a higher frequency of enthesopathies. This was confirmed and statistically significant ($\alpha=0.05$). This demonstrates that for the study of MSM, skeletons with possible enthesopathy forming diseases must be excluded to avoid over-estimation of physical activity levels.

Keywords: musculoskeletal stress markers (MSM), enthesopathies, seronegative spondyloarthropathy, diffuse idiopathic skeletal hyperostosis (DISH), bone formers

Introduction

One of the subfields of bioarchaeology is the study of activities undertaken by our ancestors (*e.g.* Hawkey and Merbs, 1995; Kennedy, 1998; Capasso *et al.,* 1999; Jurmain, 1999). The majority of this research focuses on MSM in the upper limb bones (Hawkey, 1988; Jurmain, 1999; Molleson, 1989) because this is thought to be more "activity-specific" than changes in the lower limb which may be caused by walking. The study of activity patterns is an important field: if skeletons can be used to explore labour patterns, then the lives of individuals and groups of individuals can be studied and compared temporally, geographically and socio-economically. Key stages in human history, such as the transition from hunting and gathering to agriculture may be elucidated, as may questions concerning social status and biological sex in relationship to workload. There has been considerable research in this field, as demonstrated by the dedication of a volume of the *International Journal of Osteoarchaeology* (Kennedy, 1998). A common method used is to study the presence of, what are commonly called, musculoskeletal stress markers (MSM) in skeletal remains. MSMs can be described as bone formation and/or destruction at sites of tendon, ligament, or joint capsule attachments to bone (the clinical term for the attachment is enthesis). These abnormalities take the form of lytic lesions, bone spurs (Figs. 1-2) and the presence of woven bone at the attachment site. MSM,

however, is a loaded term; it implies the direct link between musculoskeletal stress and these abnormalities. Clinically, the term enthesopathy is used, as this lacks implied aetiology. The term enthesopathy will be used throughout this paper, except where reviewing bioarchaeological research.

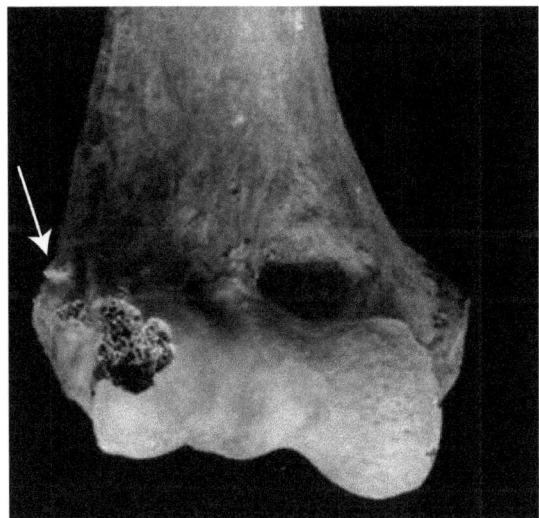

Figure 1. Example of proliferative enthesopathy (bone spur) at the lateral epicondyle (common extensor origin) of the humerus.

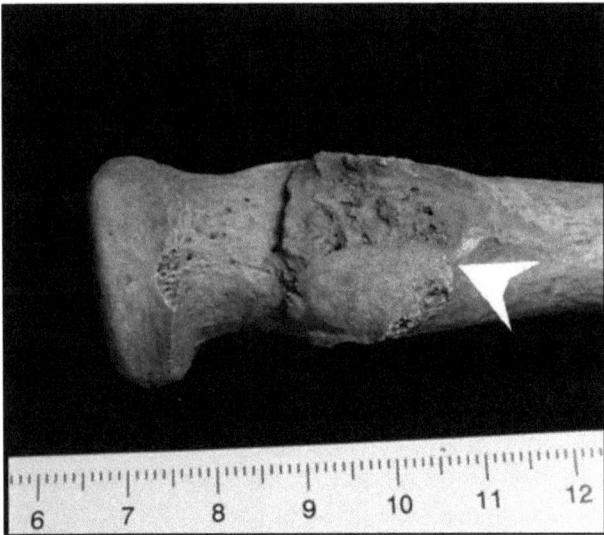

Figure 2. Example of destructive enthesopathy at the bicipital tuberosity of the radius (*biceps brachii* insertion).

Clinical research linking enthesopathies with repetitive stress does exist, but in general it focuses on their association with disease processes (particularly those in the seronegative spondyloarthropathies category). There are also bioarchaeological papers which explore these diseases (Rothschild *et al.*, 1999; Rothschild and Behman 2005) but, compared to the number published on MSM, they seem insignificant. In modern populations some of these diseases have comparatively high prevalence rates (for the seronegative spondyloarthropathies, for example, this has been estimated as 0.3% [Lories *et al.*, 2005; Saraux *et al.*, 2005]). Diffuse idiopathic skeletal hyperostosis (DISH) has a prevalence of 3%-6% in modern populations over the age of forty (Mazières and Rovensky, 2000). These diseases are not reported in this frequency in palaeopathological literature. It is possible that the manifestations of these diseases have changed over time, or that current palaeopathological diagnostic criteria rely on "classic" case descriptions and therefore cannot be relied upon to record less exuberant manifestations. This is not only a consideration for palaeopathology; clinically there is a move to recognise more unusual manifestations of seronegative spondyloarthropathy (Boyer *et al.*, 1997; Dougades *et al.*, 1991). For this reason it was decided that new recording criteria were required in palaeopathology using clinical literature. These criteria were based on the new clinical diagnostic criteria for the seronegative spondyloarthropathies, as well as, clinical literature on skeletal involvement in other enthesopathy forming diseases. The aim of this study was to test the hypothesis that skeletons fulfilling the diagnostic criteria for 'boneforming' diseases (diseases which cause bone changes at entheses, not the definition as given in Rogers *et al.*, 1997) had a significantly higher frequency of upper limb enthesopathies than those with no discernable enthesopathy-forming disease.

Materials and methods

Clinical literature on enthesopathy formation was reviewed. This included literature on enthesopathy formation caused by physical stress (Sadat-Ali, 1998), but primarily focused on disease related enthesopathy formation. Criteria to rule out possible disease-related enthesopathy formation were created based on this clinical literature. Diseases more frequently discussed in the clinical literature in relation to enthesopathy formation include the seronegative spondyloarthropathies (ankylosing spondylitis). These are a spectrum of arthropathies comprised of the following diseases: ankylosing spondylitis, Reiter's syndrome (also called reactive arthritis), psoriatic arthritis, some forms of enteropathic arthritis (arthritis associated with some diseases of the bowel, such as Crohn's disease and ulcerative colitis), some forms of juvenile chronic arthritis, and undifferentiated spondyloarthropathy. These diseases have several common features, but primarily they are not associated with rheumatoid factors in the blood serum (hence the name seronegative) and they are associated with enthesopathy formation (particularly in the spine) (Resnick and Niwayama, 1995). These diseases occur as a spectrum, and many patients do not fit into the "pigeon-holes" described above (Fournié, 2004). Consequently, these diseases are under-diagnosed in clinical medicine (Boyer *et al.*, 1997). Recent clinical research has created new diagnostic criteria for these diseases based on the spectrum of changes found in all the seronegative spondyloarthropathies (Dougades *et al.*, 1991). Some of these criteria are applicable to human skeletal remains and these form the basis of the criteria used in this study to identify possible cases of 'boneforming' diseases.

However, many of the diseases that have been linked with enthesopathy formation in clinical studies are comparatively rare, for example, POEMS (Polyneuropathy, Organomegaly, Endocrinopathy, M-protein and Skin Changes) syndrome. This disease is a plasma cell dyscrasia and, although the name highlights the non-skeletal changes associated with this disease, it is associated with skeletal changes in 97% of cases (Dispenzieri *et al.*, 2003). These manifestations include proliferative enthesopathies (Resnick, 1988). However, only a few hundred cases of this disease have been described (Rehmus and Kimball, 2005). Other diseases, such as Behçet's disease which primarily affects individuals of Middle Eastern, Near Eastern and North African ancestry (Evereklioglu, 2005), were thought to be unlikely to occur in the skeletal sample studied. Although it is unlikely that these diseases would occur in the skeletal sample studied, it was decided not to rule them out as this would have defeated the purpose of this study. Some diseases only rarely involve enthesopathy formation *e.g.* Lyme disease (Lawson and Steere, 1985). In these cases it is possible that enthesopathy formation is not associated with the disease itself, but part of an unrelated process (such as musculoskeletal stress). However, enthesopathies have been recorded in association with these diseases in the clinical literature;

consequently, recording criteria based on the clinical manifestations of these diseases were also included.

Common and rare enthesopathy forming diseases are listed in Table 1. The common location of appendicular enthesopathies is listed, along with their type: either proliferative (*e.g.* bone spurs, see Fig.1) or degenerative (*e.g.* lytic changes, such as pitting, see Fig. 2) where known. Synovial joint changes (and common locations) along with other skeletal changes are also listed. The recording criteria used for this study are summarised in Table 2. Unfortunately, many of the diagnostic criteria used clinically cannot be used on skeletal material, for example, patient histories, soft tissue changes and blood tests. This is a major limitation for these criteria.

Skeletons from the late medieval (14th-15th century) site of Fishergate House, York were used for this study. In total there were 244 inhumations, just under half of these were subadults the other half was composed of an almost equal number of males (20%) and females (21%) (Holst, 2005). Although forty-nine male skeletons were identified by Holst (this number does not include probable males), only forty-one were included in this study. Those excluded had poor preservation of the bones of the upper limb. Females were not used to avoid complicating the study with sex based hormone differences, which may alter enthesopathy expression and bias results. Burial practice and skeletal and dental evidence indicate that these skeletons all represent a low socio-economic group (Holst, 2005) and by implication this may indicate that these individuals were primarily involved in manual work. A previous study on these skeletons (Henderson, 2002) discovered that the males in this sample were robust and many had enthesopathies. Holst (2005) has also described the activity-related changes in these skeletons. These include weapon injuries, degenerative joint disease (both spinal and extraspinal), Schmorl's nodes, and MSM. It is well-known that enthesopathy prevalence increases with age. This causes a serious problem. Currently, macroscopic ageing techniques for adults are not highly accurate and they are mostly based on the degenerative changes that occur at symphyseal joints, such as the auricular surface and the pubic symphysis. These joints, like the entheses used in this study, are covered (or partially covered) in fibrocartilage and it is likely that the same biological factors involved in the ageing process affect both joints and entheses at the same rate. For this reason it was decided that the age of the adults would be defined as follows: if late fusing epiphyses have not fused or have recently fused (in which case a line is visible at the site of fusion) then the skeletons are defined as "young" adult all other skeletons are defined as "mature" adults. No further age categories were defined. Only two skeletons were found in the young category, consequently, age was not used to subdivide the skeletons. It should be noted that both of these skeletons occurred in group 1.

The entheses used in this study are all fibrocartilaginous. In skeletal remains this means that "normal" entheses have a smooth and well-delimited surface, very similar to joints covered in hyaline cartilage. Enthesopathies are defined in this study as either new bone formation or lytic lesions. New bone formation can take the form of woven bone, bone spurs (Fig. 1) or the presence of cortical bone instead of subchondral bone at an enthesis. Destructive lesions can take the form of porosity across all or part of the enthesis, or as single lytic defects. These latter are visually the same as osteochondritis dissecans and it is possible that they have a similar aetiology.

To determine whether skeletons had a 'boneforming' disease (Table 2), enthesopathy presence and lesion type (as defined above) was noted and described in the following locations: sacroiliac joint, and entheses and joint capsule attachments in the spine (Fig. 3 example of anterior longitudinal ligament ossification in the spine). Any abnormalities of phalanges, metacarpals, carpals, metatarsals and tarsals were recorded and described. Abnormalities expected were distal phalangeal tuft resorption and lytic lesions marginal to the joints or on the joints of the bones of the hands and wrists. Note that because of poor preservation of bones of the hands and feet, criteria involving the use of these bones could not be applied. Skeletons were then subdivided into two categories:

1) No signs of disease-related enthesopathy formation (normal) as listed in Table 2.
2) Fulfilling the criteria in Table 2, so presenting possible presence of disease-related enthesopathy formation and, for the purpose of brevity, called 'boneformers'. Note that this is not the general meaning of boneformer as defined by Rogers and colleagues (1997).

In order to explore activity related enthesopathy formation in the upper limb, ten upper limb entheses were recorded. These entheses were: the insertion sites of *supraspinatus, infraspinatus, teres minor, subscapularis, biceps brachii, triceps brachii* and *brachialis*; and the *anconeus*, common extensor and common flexor origins. Enthesopathies at these sites were recorded using the same methodology described above. However, for the purposes of this study only the presence or absence of an enthesopathy was recorded (and whether the site itself could be recorded). Further analysis is required to determine whether there is a different pattern of enthesopathy formation in 'boneformers' compared to those caused by physical stress.

The frequency of enthesopathies at these sites was analysed by category (*i.e.* normal and 'boneformer'). Chi-square tests ($p<0.05$) were used to compare the frequency of enthesopathy formation between categories. As stated in the introduction, the proposed hypothesis was that 'boneformers' would have a higher frequency of enthesopathy than the "normal" sample for all entheses studied. Left and right sides were pooled. Although it could be argued that left and right sides are not independent, it is likely that the physical stress experienced by left and right sides of one individual will be different. This not only means that enthesopathies

Table 1. List of diseases reviewed (based on clinical literature listed in the references) and their skeletal manifestations. Reference provided if only one source of description found.

Disease	Enthesopathy location	Joint involvement	Other skeletal involvement
Seronegative Spondylo-arthropathies	Proliferative: Any, but particularly, calcaneus (and other appendicular sites), spinal ligament entheses	Asymmetric oligoarthritis, appendicular apophyseal joint abnormalities.	Sacroiliitis, pencil-in-cup phalangeal deformity
DISH	Proliferative: Anterior longitudinal ligament (spine), any appendicular enthesis particularly pelvis, calcaneus, tarsals, olecranon of ulna, and patella	Preservation of vertebral disc space	If sacroiliitis occurs there is no intra-articular ankylosis
Fluorosis	Proliferative: Any	Vertebral body osteophytes	Osteosclerosis, periosteal bone thickening, change in bone density.
Lyme Disease	Proliferative: Enthesitis occurs, but enthesopathy is rare	Inflammatory monoarthritis typically of the knee, or less commonly degenerative joint disease	None
Ochronosis	Proliferative: Pelvis, calcaneus, femoral trochanters. Degenerative: any	Paucity of osteophyte formation, calcification of vertebral disc, large joint involvement	Blackening of cartilages
Acromegaly	Proliferative: Calcaneus, patella, femoral trochanters, tuberosities of the humerus, and entheses on the clavicle.	Widening of joint space with osteophytes (typically knee, hip and shoulder)	Cranial and hand/foot hypertrophy. Endochondral bone formation at bone cartilage junctions
Ossifying Diatheses	Proliferative: any	Generalised osteophyte formation	None reported
Leprosy	Proliferative: plantar fascia enthesis on calcaneus (Carpintero –Benítez *et al.*, 1996)	Ankylosis of joints; destruction of joints	Destructive bone changes of the hand and foot bones
Hyperpara-thyroidism	Degenerative: femoral trochanters, ischial tuberosities, humeral tuberosities, calcaneus, inferior clavicle surface, proximal ulna	Erosive arthropathy of small joints of hand and wrist (Lioté and Orcel, 2000).	Long bone curvature, cortical thinning (particularly phalanges); osteitis fibrosa cystica (Rubin and Silverberg, 2000) and bone loss (Potts, 2005)
Hypopara-thyroidism	Proliferative: Posterior paraspinal ligaments, pelvis	Apophyseal joint calcification, intervertebral disc space preservation	None reported
Hypo-thyroidism	Reported as a disease involving enthesopathy formation by Cush and Lipsky (2001)	None reported	None reported
Behçet's Disease	Enthesopathy, not linked necessarily to affected joints	Knees, ankles, hands, elbows – either monoarthritis or oligoarthritis. This can be erosive	Terminal phalanx tuft atrophy (hand)
POEMS syndrome	Proliferative: any. Especially posterior spine	None reported	Sclerosis, clubbing of fingers
X-linked Hypo-phosphatemia	Proliferative: any	None reported	Short stature, rickets, osteomalacia, fractures

Table 2. General diagnostic criteria for disease-related enthesopathy formation based on descriptions in Table 1.

Criteria	General signs	Description
1) The combination of these changes (as found typically in the seronegative spondyloarthropathies)	Spinal enthesopathy formation	Occurring at any enthesis
	Sacroiliac joint lesions	Ankylosis, erosion of joint surface, adjacent ligament ossification
2) Due to poor preservation of hand and foot bones, these two signs could not be used in this study on their own.	Phalangeal deformity	*e.g.* pencil-in-cup appearance, or distal phalangeal tuft deformity
	Erosive arthropathy of hand or wrist	
3) Signs of fluorosis	Abnormal bone density and osteosclerosis	Radiographic increase in bone density, enthesis ossification, particularly in interosseous ligaments
4) Signs of ochronosis	Blackened cartilage	Intervertebral disc space narrowing; accumulation of homogentisic acid in cartilage
5) Signs of acromegaly	Cranial hypertrophy	Enlarged mandible and long bones elongated and thickened
6) Signs of leprosy (see also phalangeal deformity)	Rhino-maxillary destruction	Ankylosis and destruction of the hand and foot bones with rhino-maxillary bone destruction

formed by physical stress will differ in their expression between the sides, it also means that disease related enthesopathy expression will probably differ between left and right sides. This is because stress is thought to be a triggering factor for enthesopathy formation in many of these diseases (Maksymowych, 2000).

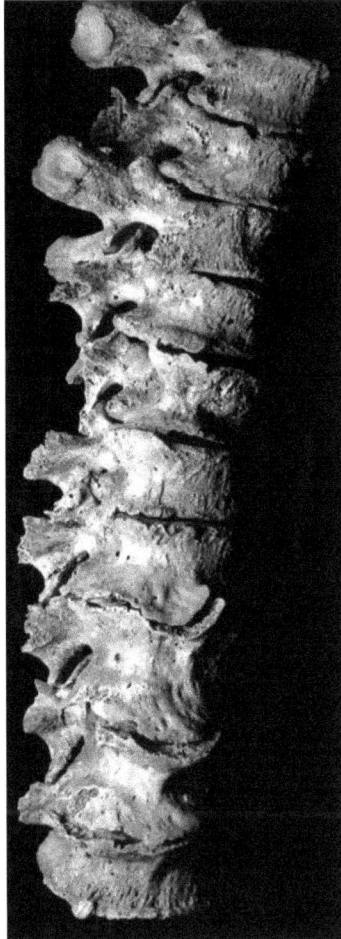

Figure 3. Spinal ligament fusion, leading to ankylosis of the spine. Skeleton F92, Fishergate House, York, England.

Results

Twenty-six skeletons were found to be normal, *i.e.* not fulfilling the criteria in Table 2 (note that criterion 2 was not utilised because too many skeletons had missing phalanges and other bones of the hands and feet, see Table 2). Eleven were found to have possible boneforming diseases, *i.e.* a combination of sacroiliac joint changes and spinal enthesopathies. No cases of leprosy, ochronosis, acromegaly, or fluorosis were found. Some skeletons exhibited changes in the small bones of the hands and feet, which were recorded but not used to group the skeletons. Eight skeletons were too poorly preserved to observe either the sacroiliac joints or the spine and were excluded from the study.

Table 3 presents the frequency of enthesopathies seen in each group. Four of the 'boneformers' were diagnosed with DISH or possible seronegative spondyloarthropathy

by Holst (2005). The other skeletons had combinations of spinal ligament and sacroiliac joint ossification, but no definite disease could be diagnosed. Figure 4 demonstrates that the frequency of enthesopathies was consistently higher in the 'boneformers'. As can be seen in this figure, fewer enthesopathies occurred in the "normal" category than in the 'boneformers'. Chi-square tests demonstrated that there was a significantly higher frequency ($p<0.001$) of enthesopathies in the 'boneformers'. Table 4 presents the significance for each enthesis. It should be noted that small sample sizes caused by poor preservation, particularly in the rotator cuff, may have had an effect on the results.

Table 3. Frequency of enthesopathies observed in the upper limb bones (left and right sides pooled).

Enthesis	Non-boneformers (26 skeletons) no. affected (%)	Boneformers (11 skeletons) no. affected (%)
Supraspinatus	9/34 (26%)	5/6 (83%)
Common extensor origin	22/39 (56%)	14/15 (93%)
Subscapularis	26/35 (74%)	8/11 (73%)
Infraspinatus	17/36 (47%)	5/6 (83%)
Teres minor	10/32 (31%)	4/6 (67%)
Anconeus	10/40 (25%)	8/14 (57%)
Common flexor origin	12/41 (29%)	13/17 (76%)
Biceps brachii	23/39 (59%)	11/13 (85%)
Triceps brachii	11/41 (27%)	12/19 (63%)
Brachialis	13/44 (30%)	13/19 (68%)

Table 4. Chi-square tests comparing the frequency of enthesopathies at different entheses between 'boneformers' and 'normal' skeletons.

Enthesis	Significant difference in frequency	Comment
Subscapularis	-	Frequency of enthesopathies higher in the non-boneformers (see Fig. 4). $p=0.9182$
Supraspinatus	X	$p=0.0071$
Infraspinatus	-	$p=0.1011$
Teres minor	-	$p=0.0989$
Common extensor origin	X	$p=0.0074$
Anconeus	X	$p=0.0281$
Common flexor origin	X	$p=0.0010$
Triceps brachii	X	$p=0.0071$
Brachialis	X	$p=0.0040$
Biceps brachii	-	$p=0.0924$

X = statistically significant ($p<0.05$); - = not significant ($p>0.05$)

Discussion

The primary goal of bioarchaeology is the reconstruction of the everyday lives of people who lived in the past through the analysis of their skeletal remains. MSM are bone forming or bone destroying changes at the sites of soft tissue attachments, *e.g.* muscles and ligaments, to bone. These soft tissues are those that act upon the bones

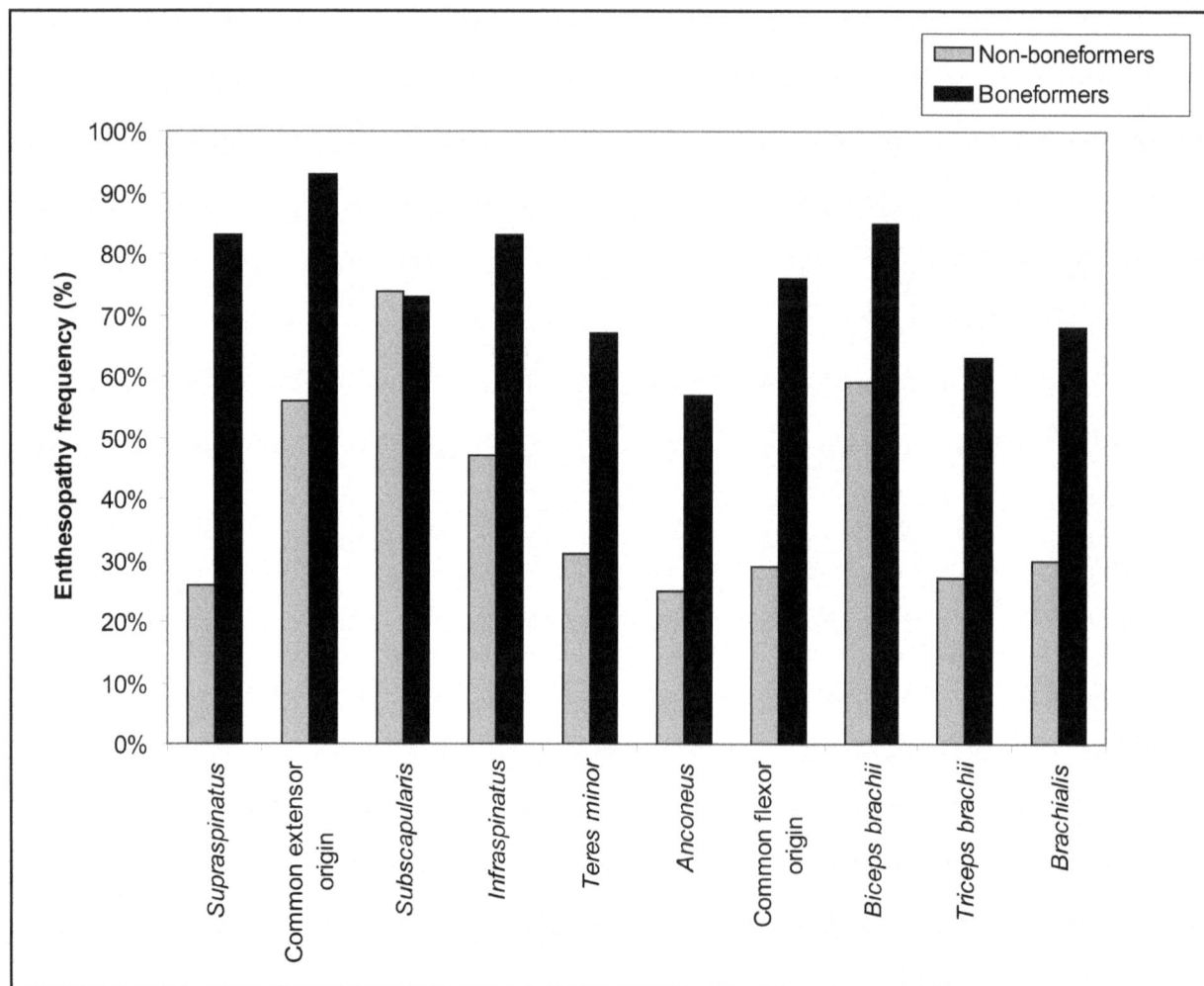

Figure 4. Enthesopathy frequency by skeleton category (*i.e.* 'boneformers' as opposed to 'non-boneformers').

of the skeleton to move it, or stabilise it during movement. For this reason the changes at these sites are thought to be related to physical stress, such as muscle overloading, and the location of the abnormality is believed to indicate the direction of the physical stress acting on the skeleton. If the relationship between physical stress and abnormality is this simple, then the study of MSM holds huge potential for research into activity-related stress in human skeletal assemblages. However, a study of clinical literature has highlighted the number of diseases associated with enthesopathy formation. It has also demonstrated the requirement to examine whether skeletons with possible enthesopathy forming diseases had a statistically significant increased frequency of upper limb enthesopathies. Determining this is critical. If there is a link between 'boneforming' diseases and an increased frequency of upper limb enthesopathies, then it is clear that not all enthesopathies should be recorded or interpreted as indicators of repetitive physical stress and that doing so could overestimate the activity-levels in skeletal samples.

It was hypothesised, based on the clinical literature, that there would be a higher frequency of enthesopathies in the upper limb in individuals fulfilling the criteria for possible disease presence than those with no signs of

these diseases. The results demonstrate this and that it is statistically significant ($p<0.05$). All entheses, except the *subscapularis* insertion demonstrated higher frequencies of enthesopathies in 'boneformers' than in the normal skeletons, and in the majority of cases this was a statistically significant difference (Table 4). It is unclear why the *subscapularis* insertion did not conform to this model. It may be a reflection of sample size. However, it is noteworthy that the *subscapularis* insertion often demonstrates higher than expected rates of enthesopathy formation (Chapman, 1997; Henderson, 2005; Henderson and Villotte, in prep.). Clinical literature indicates that the *supraspinatus* insertion should be the most affected in the upper limb, because rotator cuff tears are thought to begin in and spread from this tendon (Pollock *et al.*, 1995). This is supported by magnetic resonance imaging of the rotator cuff (Lambert *et al.*, 2004). It is as yet unclear, why these contradictory data exist. It is possible that the *supraspinatus* is most affected by soft tissue damage of a type which does not alter the enthesis, whereas the damage to the *subscapularis* occurs at or adjacent to the insertion site, thereby modifying it. Further research is required.

It should be noted that the diagnostic criteria used in this study cannot be used to diagnose the individual diseases, because the relationship between the diagnostic criteria used in this study and actual disease presence has not been researched. It is also possible that individual skeletons with these diseases, but not fulfilling the criteria set out in Table 2, have 'slipped through the net', because of the lack of soft tissue and clinical history required to diagnose these diseases clinically. Some clinical studies indicate that enthesopathy formation can be the first sign of these diseases (Marzo-Ortega, 2002) and furthermore, that there is a relationship between the seronegative spondyloarthropathies and biomechanical stress (McGonagle *et al.,* 2001). Differentiating between these cases and those with enthesopathies caused by musculoskeletal stress is currently impossible. Further advances in clinical medicine are required before this can be attempted by bioarchaeologists. This is a major limitation for studies of activity-related stress using MSM.

Conclusion

The aim of this study was to determine whether there was a higher frequency of enthesopathies in the upper limb bones of skeletons with diseases associated with enthesopathy formation. The upper limb was chosen, because this is the region of the human skeleton most commonly used by bioarchaeologists to study repetitive activity-patterns. If enthesopathies can be used to study such activity-patterns then the daily lives of people in the past can be better understood. To achieve this, other factors known to cause enthesopathy formation must be considered to avoid overestimating activity-levels.

It has been confirmed by this study that there are numerous diseases associated with enthesopathy formation. The comparison of skeletons with and without skeletal signs of these diseases demonstrated an increase in enthesopathy frequency for the entheses studied in those with possible 'boneforming' diseases. This study has obvious limitations: firstly, the reliance on purely skeletal remains makes the diagnosis of these diseases difficult. It should be remembered that these are only criteria designed to highlight possible cases of disease-related enthesopathy formation; they are not diagnostic criteria for any of the diseases discussed. Secondly, cases in which soft tissue changes are the sole manifestation of the disease cannot be recognised in skeletal remains. Consequently, it is possible that individuals have been categorised incorrectly. However, if enthesopathies are to be utilised by bioarchaeologists to study activity-related stress, then the necessity for stringent criteria to rule out enthesopathies with different aetiologies is the key to preventing over-diagnosis of activity-related enthesopathies and misinterpretation of activity levels in skeletal remains.

Acknowledgements

Thanks are due to the following individuals and organisations: The Institute of Bioarchaeology for financial support enabling me to attend the 8th Annual BABAO conference in Birmingham, 15th-17th of September, 2006; Professor C. A. Roberts and Dr. A. R. Millard for feedback and support during my PhD; M. Holst (originally from Field Archaeology Specialists), for the skeletal analysis and M. Griffiths Associates, the consultant for the excavation Fishergate House, York, by Field Archaeology Specialists.

This work is part of ongoing research for a PhD

Literature cited

Boyer, G.S., Templin, D.W., Bowler, A., Lawrence, R.C., Everett, D.F., Heyse, S.P., Cornoni-Huntley, J. and Goring, W.P. 1997. "A comparison of patients with spondyloarthropathy seen in specialty clinics with those identified in a communitywide epidemiologic study: has the classic case misled us?" *Archives of Internal Medicine* 157: 2111-2117.

Capasso L., Kennedy, K.A.R., Wilczak, C.A. 1999. *Atlas of Occupational Markers on Human Remains.* Teramo, Italy: Edigrafital S.p.A.

Carpintero-Benítez, P., Logroño, C. and Collantes-Estevez, E. 1996. "Enthesopathy in Leprosy." *Journal of Rheumatology* 23: 1020-1021.

Chapman, N.E.M. 1997. "Evidence for Spanish Influence on Activity Induced Musculoskeletal Stress Markers at Pecos Pueblo." *International Journal of Osteoarchaeology* 7: 497-506.

Cush, J. and Lipsky, P.E. 2001. "Reiter's Syndrome and Reactive Arthritis". In: Koopman, W. J. (ed.) *Arthritis and Allied Conditions.* Philadelphia: Lippincott Williams and Wilkins. 1: 1324-1344.

Dispenzieri, A., Kyle, R.A., Lacy, M.Q., Rajkumar, S.V., Therneau, T.M., Larson, D.R., Greipp, P.R., Witzig, T.E., Basu, R., Suarez, G.A., Fonseca, R., Lust, J.A. and Gertz, M.A. 2003. "POEMS syndrome: definitions and long-term outcome." *Blood* 101: 2496-2506.

Dougades, M., van der Linden, S., Juhlin, R., Huitfeldt, B., Amor, B., Calin, A., Cats, A., Dijkmans, B., Olivieri, I., Pasero, G., Veys, E. and Zeidler, H. 1991. "The European Spondyloarthropathy Study Group Preliminary Criteria for the Classification of Spondyloarthropathy." *Arthritis and Rheumatism* 34: 1218-1227.

Evereklioglu, C. 2005. "Current concepts in the etiology and treatment of Behçet disease." *Survey of Ophthalmology* 50: 297-350.

Fournié, B. 2004. "Pathology and clinico-pathologic correlations in spondyloarthropathies." *Joint Bone Spine* 71: 525-529.

Hawkey, D.E. 1988 "Use of Upper Extremity Enthesopathies to Indicate Habitual Activity Patterns" M.A. Arizona State University.

Hawkey, D.E., and Merbs, C.F. 1995. "Activity-induced Musculoskeletal Stress Markers (MSM) and Subsistence Strategy Changes among Ancient Hudson Bay Eskimos". *International Journal of Osteoarchaeology* 5: 324-338.

Henderson, C.Y. 2002 "Are the presence or absence of post-cranial nonmetric traits linked to occupation and lifestyle?" MSc dissertation. Durham. University of Durham.

Henderson, C.Y. 2005. "Measuring Rotator Cuff Disease". Paper presented at the Paleopathology Association, 32nd Annual North America Meeting, Milwaukee, Wisconsin.

Henderson, C.Y. and Villotte, S. in prep. "An Anatomical Approach to Musculoskeletal Stress Markers: Preliminary Results".

Holst, M. 2005 "Artefacts and Environmental Evidence: Human Bone. Summary of Skeletal Analysis". In Spall, C.A. and Toop, N.J. (eds.) *Blue Bridge Lane and Fishergate House, York. Report on Excavations: July 2000 to July 2002.* Archaeological Planning Consultancy Ltd.

Jurmain, R.D. 1999. *Stories from the Skeleton: Behavioural Reconstruction in Human Osteology.* Amsterdam: Gordon and Breach.

Kennedy, K.A.R. 1998. "Markers of Occupational Stress: Conspectus and Prognosis of Research" *International Journal of Osteoarchaeology* 8: 305-310.

Lambert, R.G.W., Dhillon, S.S., Jhangri, G.S., Sacks, J., Sacks, H., Wong, B., Russell, A.S. and Maksymowych, W.P. 2004. "High Prevalence of Symptomatic Enthesopathy of the Shoulder in Ankylosing Spondylitis: Deltoid Origin Involvement Constitutes a Hallmark of Disease." *Arthritis and Rheumatism* 51: 681-690.

Lawson, J.P. and Steere, A.C. 1985. "Lyme Arthritis: Radiologic Findings." *Radiology* 154: 37-43.

Lioté, F. and Orcel, P. 2000. "Osteoarticular disorders of endocrine origin." *Ballière's Clinical Rheumatology* 14: 251-276.

Lories, R.J.U, Derese, I., and Luyten, F.P. 2005. "Modulation of bone morphogenetic protein signaling inhibits the onset and progression of ankylosing enthesitis." *Journal of Clinical Investigation* 115: 1571-1579.

Maksymowych, W.P. 2000. "Ankylosing Spondylitis -At the Interface of Bone and Cartilage [editorial]" *The Journal of Rheumatology* 27: 2295-2301.

Marzo-Ortega, H., Emery, P. and McGonagle, D. 2002. "The Concept of Disease Modification in Spondyloarthropathy." *The Journal of Rheumatology* 29: 1583-1585.

Mazières, B., and Rovensky, J. 2000. "Non-inflammatory enthesopathies of the spine a diagnostic approach". *Ballière's Clinical Rheumatology* 14: 201-217.

McGonagle, D., Stockwin, L., Isaac, J. and Emery, P. 2001. "An Enthesitis Based Model for the Pathogenesis of Spondyloarthropathy. Additive Effects of Microbial Adjuvant and Biomechanical Factors at Disease Sites (editorial)." *The Journal of Rheumatology* 28: 2155-2159.

Molleson, T. 1989 "Seed preparation in the Mesolithic: the osteological evidence" *Antiquity.* 63: 356-362.

Pollock, R.G., Flatow, E.L., Bigliani, L.U., Kelkar, R. and Mow, V.C. 1995. "Shoulder Biomechanics and Repetitive Motion". In: Gordon, S.L., Blair, S.J. and Fine, L.J. (eds.) *Repetitive Motion Disorders of the Upper Extremity.* Rosemont, Illinois: American Academy of Orthopaedic Surgeons. 145-160.

Potts, J. T. 2005. "Parathyroid hormone: past and present." *Journal of Endocrinology* 187: 311–325.

Rehmus, W. and Kimball, A.B. 2005. "POEMS syndrome".http://www.emedicine.com/derm/topic771.htm. (Accessed November 2006).

Resnick, D. 1988. Plasma Cell Dyscrasias and Dysgammaglobulinemias. In: Resnick D. and Niwayama G. (eds.) *Diagnosis of Bone and Joint Disorders.* Philadelphia: W.B. Saunders Company. 2358-2403.

Resnick, D. and Niwayama, G. 1995. "Rheumatoid Arthritis and the Seronegative Spondyloarthropathies: Radiographic and Pathologic Concepts". In: Resnick, D. (ed.) *Diagnosis of Bone and Joint Disorders.* Philadelphia: W B Saunders Company. Vol. 2: 807-865.

Rogers, J., Shepstone, L. and Dieppe, P. 1997. "Bone formers: osteophyte and enthesophyte formation are positively associated" *Annals of the Rheumatic Diseases* 56: 85-90.

Rothschild, B.M., Arriaza, B. Woods, RJ. and Dutour, O. 1999. "Spondyloarthropathy identified as the etiology of Nubian erosive arthritis." *American Journal of Physical Anthropology* 109: 259-267.

Rothschild, B.M. and Behman, S. 2005. "The often overlooked digital tuft: clues to diagnosis and pathophysiology of neuropathic disease and spondyloarthropathy." *Annals of the Rheumatic Diseases* 64: 286-290.

Rubin, M. R. and Silverberg, S.J. 2000. "Rheumatic manifestations of primary hyperparathyroidism and parathyroid hormone therapy." *Current Rheumatology reports* 4: 179-185.

Sadat-Ali, M. 1998. "Plantar Fasciitis/Calcaneal Spur among Security Forces Personnel". *Military Medicine* 163: 56-57.

Saraux, A., Guillemin, F., Guggenbuhl, P., Roux, C.H., Fardellone, P., Le Bihan, E., Cantagrel, A., Chary-Valckenaere, I., Euller-Ziegler, L., Flipo, R.M., Juvin, R., Behier, J.M., Fautrel, B., Masson, C. and Coste, J. 2005. "Prevalence of spondyloarthropathies in France" *Annals of the Rheumatic Diseases* 64: 1431-5.

Determination of useful incision mark characteristics for microscopic forensic analysis

Catherine Tennick, Jennie Robinson and Micheal Wysocki

School of Forensic and Investigative Sciences, UCLAN,
Preston, Lancashire, PR1 2HE
e-mail address for correspondence: cjtennick@uclan.ac.uk

Abstract

Cut mark analysis to date has been intermittently and superficially researched across a range of disciplines, despite its potential to significantly contribute to criminal investigation. Decomposition and liquefaction of tissues may prevent conventional pathological analysis to determine weapon type, and therefore examination of trauma to remaining bone tissue may be necessary.

Optical Microscopy was used to examine knife cuts on fleshed porcine bone. Incised cuts were made by a range of serrated, scalloped and fine-edged blades, resulting in 250 observable cuts for examination. A review of existing literature was undertaken to compile a scoring system which would allow accurate and reliable information about cut marks to be recorded, and to determine whether documented characteristics from existing archaeological research could be readily applied to forensic analysis. Observable cut mark characteristics are defined, and a number of significant relationships established, indicating that aspects of archaeological observation of stone and bone tools can also be successfully applied to the analysis of metal knife blades.

Keywords: sharp force trauma, microscopy, cut marks, weapon identification

Introduction

The pathological analysis of flesh wounds can establish weapon type by wound shape, edge characteristics, and rarely, by comparison of a blade with remaining fragments in soft tissue (Adelson, 1974; DiMaio and DiMaio, 1993). The identification of sharp force trauma (SFT) on human skeletal remains is also important in medicolegal cases; however, the absence of soft tissue prevents conventional wound analysis techniques. Microscopy has been successfully used in toolmark examination, but has rarely been applied to processes such as SFT on bone in forensic casework (Houck, 1998). Cut mark analysis to date has been intermittently examined across a range of disciplines, despite its potential to significantly contribute to criminal investigation (Symes *et al.*, 2002). There are few published works with a forensic perspective related to incision marks made on bone and the research already carried out is limited in its scope and application; the available literature is widely scattered throughout a number of different fields and across several decades. This includes archaeology (Wenham, 1989; Blumenshine *et al.*, 1996; Greenfield, 1999; Smith and Brickley, 2004; Loe and Cox 2005), paleoanthropology (Bunn 1981; Potts and Shipman, 1981; Shipman and Rose, 1983; Bromage and Boyde, 1984; Eickhoff and Herrmann, 1985; Olsen, 1988; Shipman and Rose, 1988) and forensic science (Houck, 1998; Bartelink *et al.*, 2001; Alunni Perret *et al.*, 2005)

As time since death increases, the amount of remaining evidence associated with human remains decreases. The rigidity of bone means that the dimensions and shapes of wounds are better maintained than in skin and other soft tissues (Spitz, 1993:287) and therefore cut marks on bone may provide viable diagnostic evidence for a much longer *post mortem* period than other evidence types. Current data shows that sharp instruments are the most frequent cause of homicidal deaths in the UK (Coleman *et al.*, 2006). Despite this knife wound analysis to date has been insufficient, and as an area of research inadequately addressed (Symes *et al.*, 2002:405).

Current knowledge.

Despite the sparse availability of forensic literature, cut mark analysis in other disciplines such as archaeology and paleoanthropology is more widely researched. Much of the literature examines stone and bone tools, although some later papers do examine metal blades also (Olsen, 1988; Wenham, 1989; Blumenschine *et al.*, 1996; Greenfield, 1999). Many of the observations and principles behind the examination of archaeological tools may be transferable to the forensic analysis of metal blade marks. Shipman and Rose (1983: 66) observed that some marks exhibited features related to the morphology of the tools that made them. Olsen (1988: 343) also noted that parallel striae from different marks made by the same tool could sometimes be matched. This potential for identification is exactly what the forensic investigator is interested in when trying to establish whether a particular object made characteristic marks recovered from a crime scene.

Class and individual characteristics

Prieto (2007) acknowledges that when bone is sectioned or crossed by a weapon, it can reveal more conclusive details about weapon characteristics than soft tissue

Table 1. An overview of selected papers detailing observed characteristics of cut marks.

Authors	Date	Toolmark type	Microscopic analysis		Observed/ Suggested characteristics of cut marks								
			SEM	Low power	Width	Depth	Striae	Wall and Edge Morphology	Cross-section shape	Smear/ Chip/ Fault	Floor	Shoulder effect/ Barbs	Lateral Ridging
Potts and Shipman	1981	Stone	✓				✓		✓				
Bunn	1981	Stone							✓				
Shipman and Rose	1983 1988	Bone Stone	✓		✓	✓	✓					✓	
Shipman	1983 1988	Bone Stone	✓		✓		✓	✓	✓				
Bromage and Boyde	1984	Stone Bone	✓							✓			
Eickhoff and Hermann	1985	Stone			✓	✓	✓	✓	✓				
Olsen	1988	Stone Metal	✓	Hand lens									
Wenham	1989	Metal	✓	✓			✓	✓					
Blumenschine	1996	Stone Metal		✓			✓		✓				
Houck	1998	Bone	✓				✓						
Greenfield	1998	Stone Metal	✓						✓				
Bartelink et al.	2001	Metal	✓		✓	✓							
Smith and Brickley	2004	Stone Metal	✓		✓	✓	✓		✓				
Loe and Cox	2005	Stone Metal		✓		✓	✓	✓	✓				
Alunni-Perret et al.	2006	Metal	✓		✓	✓	✓	✓	✓				✓
Tennick	2007	Metal		✓	✓	✓	✓	✓	✓		✓		✓

Barbs : Sharp point facing away from the tips of incision marks as a result of involuntary hand movements by the operator (Shipman and Rose, 1983:66)

Shoulder marks: Short marks parallel to slicing mark that are inflicted at the same time, as a result of the shoulder of the tool making contact with the bone (Shipman and Rose, 1983:66) alone. When undertaking cut mark examination, there are two types of characteristic that are pertinent for analysis; class and individual. The class characteristics of a cut mark are those that may be associated with a particular group, but never a single source, such as the ability to determine that a mark on bone was made by a metal knife rather than a stone tool. Class characteristics can become more specific depending on the number of traits considered in the examination (Houck, 1998:412). Thus class evidence has the potential to be individualising, but a unique outcome is rare. Individual characteristics therefore, are those that can be attributed to a common source with a very high degree of certainty (Saferstein, 2001: 65); this might be the determination that the mark was made by one serrated kitchen knife, and no other knife has the necessary individual characteristics to belong in this group. Individual characteristics can be largely attributed to wear and tear through repeated use of an individual knife blade (Rao and Hart, 1983).

In archaeological research, cut marks are rarely examined exclusively. Microscopic criteria have been suggested as a means to identify various unknown marks that may mimic cut marks, including: carnivore toothmarks, rodent gnawing marks, weathering, sedimentary abrasion, burning, root etching and trampling (Potts and Shipman, 1981; Shipman, 1981; Shipman, 1983; Olsen and Shipman, 1988). Cut marks have also been examined in association with scavenger toothmarks, percussion marks, and modern excavation marks (Eickhoff and Herrmann, 1985; Blumenshine *et al.*, 1996; Smith and Brickley, 2004; Loe and Cox, 2005).

Much of the research is concerned with stone and bone tools, rather than metal blades. Two studies investigate differences between metal and stone tools. Olsen (1988) conducted an experimental study with stone and knife cuts on modern bone. She suggested that distinguishing criteria are possible, and Greenfield (1999) carried out further experiments involving 12 metal blades as well as stone tools. Both studies involved examining casts or replicas of the cut in silicone, producing a negative impression.

Work by Rose (1983) on replication of samples using casting compounds, lists some of the limitations of this form of examination. These include tendencies of the casting compound to remove very small parts of the specimen's surface (Rose, 1983: 259), and the possibility of casting compound remaining in recesses of porous bone. She also states that specimens with small projections are more difficult to replicate accurately. The inherent limitations of this technique therefore make it unsuitable for the examination of very small cut marks (in the current experimental sample, the marks are typically less than 1mm wide), particularly when the purpose of forensic examination is the preservation of characteristics on bone for comparison with test marks from a suspect weapon. Whilst this is appropriate when the focus of examination may be general cut mark morphology, for forensic examination the preservation of both class and

individual characteristics that may be present in the mark is vital.

Although ultimately concerned with marks on bone, Greenfield's (1999) study used soft pine wood as a cutting medium to examine the cut mark profiles. This is because pine wood is softer than bone and more likely to accurately replicate the edge accurately in the cutting process. As a method of experimentation, it may be unsuitable for forensic analysis because, as Bromage and Boyde (1984:361) point out, the individual bone on which a cut mark is made may contribute to cut mark morphology. This is a contradiction to the findings of Shipman and Rose (1983) who found that marks remained consistent. The presumption is that the mark morphology was constant because experiments were based on one bone or one type of bone (Bromage and Boyde, 1984:361). This highlighted the need to consider the bone surface as a potential variable in any further experiments carried out.

Aims

It has been established that forensic analysis of sharp blade incision on bone has, to date, been limited. Analysis of stone and bone tool incisions has been well documented (Table 1) but metal blade incisions on bone, particularly for forensic examination, have only recently been investigated (Houck, 1998; Bartelink *et al.*, 2001; Alunni-Perret *et al.*, 2005). The purpose of this interim paper is to review existing inter-disciplinary knowledge about the observation and analysis of incision marks made by metal blades.

In order to review cut mark analysis, the knife sample size has been expanded (n.=10) beyond previous studies of forensic interest, in addition to observing a more comprehensive number of mark characteristics drawn from a series of diverse literature. Analysis of the marks (n.=250) gives an indication of which cut mark features may be useful in distinguishing between metal blade types, and whether methods considered traditionally useful in disciplines other than forensic science, can be readily applied in this field.

Methods

Cutting tools

Hunt and Cowling (1991) examined 100 homicidal stabbing cases, and report that the most frequently used weapon was a kitchen knife or carving knife (55%), possibly as a result of the ease with which they can be obtained. For the current experimental sample, ten metal blades were selected to create the incision marks on bone (Table 2). All of the sample blades are readily available kitchen knives, and the sample set can be seen in Figure 1. These consisted of three serrated kitchen (steak) knives, six fine-edged blades of varying length and size, and one scalloped blade (bread knife). Examples of each blade type can be seen in Figure 2.

Table 2. Details of knife types used in experimental incisions on bone. For images of each knife, see Figure 1.

Knife ID	Knife Description	Blade Type	Cutting Edge	New/Used
1	Steak knife, unbranded	Serrated to left	Double	Used
2	Steak knife, unbranded	Serrated to left	Double	New
3	Steak knife, unbranded	Serrated to left	Double	New
4	Chef's knife, unbranded	Fine	Single - left	Used
5	Carving knife, unbranded	Fine	Single - left	New
6	Carving knife, "Kitchen Devil" brand	Fine	Double	New
7	Chef's knife, "Kitchen Devil" brand	Fine	Double	New
8	Paring knife, "Kitchen Devil" brand	Fine	Double	New
9	Vegetable knife, "Kitchen Devil" brand	Fine	Double	New
10	Bread Knife, "Kitchen Devil" brand	Scalloped to left	Double	New

This is the largest sample of metal knife blades used on bone in a forensic experiment. Houck (1998) and Bartelink *et al*. (2001) used three knives, Alunni–Perret *et al*., (2005) used only one. In addition, all of the knives used in the study were bought new by the author. Some of the knives were unused prior to this experiment; all knives documented as 'used', have had their prior uses catalogued to provide a record of the amount of wear on each blade, for potential later comparison of the effect of wear on marks made by metal blades.

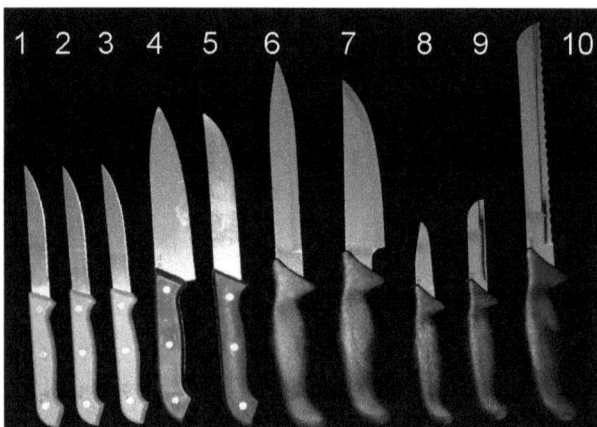

Figure 1. Knife sample set, from 1-10. For knife details, see Table 2.

Medium for examination

Porcine ribs were used, as non-human mammalian bone is considered to be a suitable medium for this type of experiment (Houck, 1998). Although some recent forensic studies have used lower-limb bones as a cutting medium (Houck, 1998; Tucker *et al.*, 2001; Alunni-Perret *et al.*, 2005), Schmidt and Pollak (2006:113) observed sharp force trauma injuries in 158 knife attack patients, and indicated that the least common location for sharp force trauma injury in 158 knife attack patients was the lower extremities (6.1%). In contrast, the thoracic area (containing the ribcage) was most frequently injured (45.9%). The suggestion that the thoracic area is a common target for stab wounds is also supported by the earlier work of Adelson (1974), Hunt and Cowling (1991), Rouse (1994) and Rogde *et al.* (2000).

In order to monitor whether the condition of the bone surface affected the morphology of the mark, observations were made of the bone surface surrounding each mark to be scored. The ribs were individual, but each remained articulated with the vertebrae, and before the marks were made the bones had approximately 5mm of adhering muscle tissue. Recent studies (Houck 1998; Alunni-Perret *et al.*, 2005) make marks directly onto bone through the periosteum. The importance of the presence of soft tissue as a shield from stone and bone tools was noted by Shipman and Rose (1983: 86), but the effect of different soft tissue thicknesses on marks made by metal blades has also been investigated. Knight (1975) stated that skin is the most resistive tissue, and once a knife penetrates skin, no further force need be applied. O'Callaghan *et al.* (1999) confirmed that skin has the highest resistance, but that muscle also demonstrates a resistive force, but it is concluded that resistance of underlying tissue is easily overcome by an assailant performing a stabbing action and is inconsequential in such cases (O'Callaghan *et al.,* 1999). The experiment undertaken by O'Callaghan *et al.,* (1999) stabbed through 10cm of skin, muscle and subcutaneous fat, therefore it is considered that the presence of several millimetres of tissue in this experiment will have a negligible effect on the resultant cut marks.

Method of application

Previous authors (Houck, 1998; Bartelink *et al.*, 2001; Alunni-Perret *et al.*, 2005) with interests in the forensic applications of cut mark analysis used mechanical application of knife blades in order to replicate marks, but mechanical application may result in artificial levels of similarity. Chadwick *et al.* (1999) carried out comparative experiments between a series of 20 volunteers and drop-tower tests (mechanical apparatus with a blade attached) stabbing a target consisting of simulated flesh covered with stab resistant material, and observed that measurable differences in energy, momentum and velocity existed between the mechanical technique and the manual volunteers. In the human stab, energy and momentum measured are made up of a number of different masses travelling at different velocities, and the mechanical drop-tower has only one mass in motion, which appears to be a limitation of using mechanical equipment when considering blade penetration as a variable (Chadwick *et al.*, 1999:42-43).

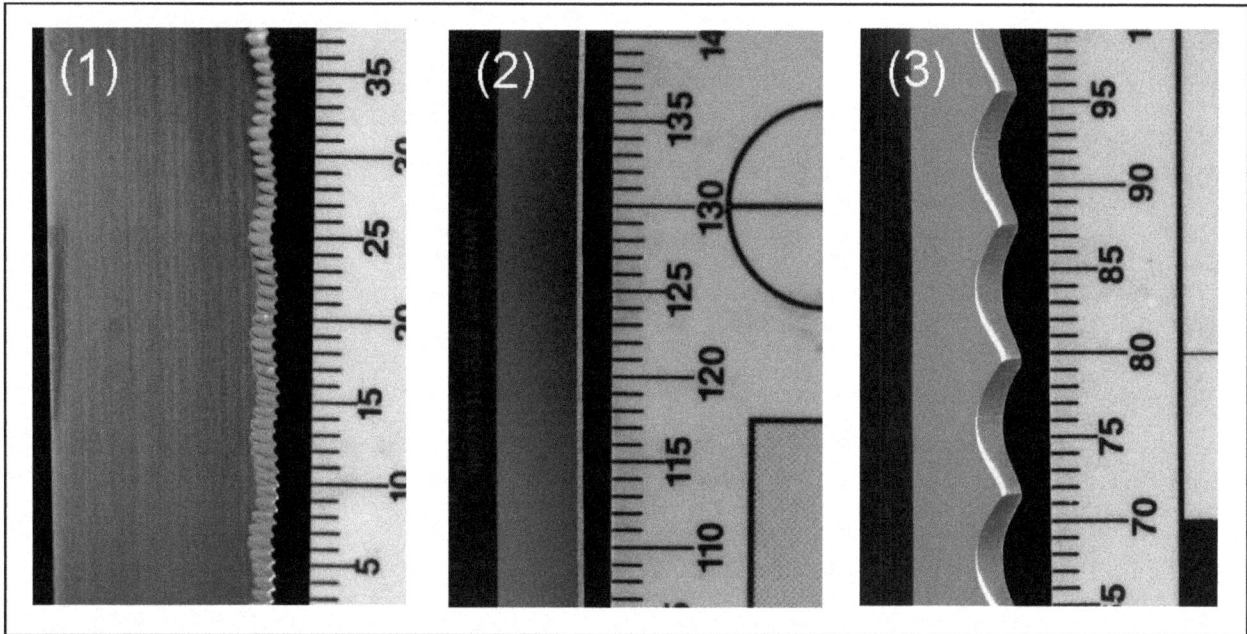

Figure 2. Typical examples of knife blade types examined: (1) Serrated, (2) Fine, (3) Scalloped.

Manual variation can be minimised by using the same operator, and ensuring the knife is held in the same position in all cases – force and angle can therefore be monitored for consistency between marks. In this case, each knife tip was lifted to shoulder height for each cut, and the knife lowered to incise the bone surface. Marks made manually that show similar features may have greater significance in practical application, as marks examined in the field could be subject to greater variation.

Twenty cuts were made on the anterior and posterior surfaces of each pig rib. The resultant marks can be categorised as incised rather than stab wounds because the marks are longer than they are deep (Adelson, 1974; Spitz, 1993). This is a model for human trauma, and therefore the analogous terms superior (anterior) and inferior (posterior) will be used in the text to describe anatomical location of the marks. Each rib contains marks representative of one knife blade.

Preparation of bone material

Preserving microscopic detail within each mark was a priority when selecting a technique for removing soft tissues from the bones. Boiling does not affect microscopic features of marks on bone (Bromage and Boyde, 1984; Shipman and Rose, 1988) although Bromage and Boyde (1984:363) did note that bones prepared in a solution of enzyme detergent showed no fine striae. Fenton *et al.* (2003) suggest a method for safe preparation of forensic skeletal remains involving enzyme detergent, but in considering the findings of Bromage and Boyde (1984), a modified technique was used. Each bone was suspended in a weak solution of enzyme detergent, simmering until the flesh was soft and

easy to remove (approximately four hours). Suspending the bones prevented the cut-marked surfaces contacting either the sides of the container or other bone surfaces, which could potentially cause damage to the cuts or the bone surface. The bones were removed from the solution, gently rinsed in water and the attached flesh was carefully removed using plastic tweezers, avoiding contact with the bone surface. The samples were then placed in a solution of distilled water which was allowed to simmer until all remaining traces of flesh and periosteum were removed from the bones.

Examination

Each mark was examined whilst fresh, using a Leica S60E Transmitted Light Stereomicroscope with a magnification range of 6.3x to 40x. The bones were placed on free-standing, moveable supports to prevent marks from lying on a hard surface. This also permitted manipulation under the microscope in order to view different aspects of the cuts, because changing the orientation of a specimen can reveal previously unobserved features (Shipman and Rose, 1983: 92).

Lengths and widths were not recorded at this stage because accurate measurements are made at magnifications of 50x or more, and callipers do not give accurate measurements for indented features like cut marks (Shipman and Rose 1983: 92). Employing the use of the scanning electron microscope will provide detailed and accurate measurement data, and this will be carried out in the next phase of work. The incident light source for low power microscopy was also systematically altered (Blumenschine *et al.*, 1996:505) in order to ensure accurate observations of any particular feature.

Scoring

The cross-disciplinary study of cut mark analysis to date has failed to produce a consistent, descriptive and accurate terminology (Symes *et al.*, 2002). Published criteria for identification of metal cut marks vary in detail and their purpose for discrimination. Little research exists in determining identification of different metal blade types, whereas many different characteristics have been identified for establishing differences between cut marks and percussion pits, or scavenger tooth marks (e.g. Blumenschine *et al.*, 1996; Loe and Cox, 2005), as well as distinguishing between different types of metal weapons (Wenham, 1989), and modern forensic studies into inter-blade characteristics (Houck, 1998; Bartelink *et al.*, 2001). It was therefore necessary to review the available literature across a range of subjects in order to identify the depth and nature of observations made by others. This was combined with the experience of preliminary observations made by the author in order to create a coherent and standardised recording method, appropriate for recording the nature of a cut mark that may be of forensic interest.

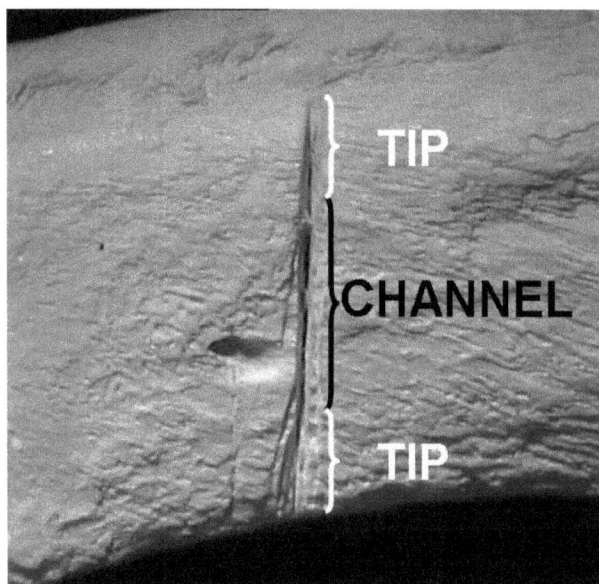

Figure 3. Fine-edged blade mark 7, imaged on a Projectina Comparison Macroscope at 105x. The kerf components are labelled.

Symes (1992) designated the channel or groove made by the action of a blade on a surface as the kerf. During mark analysis, it was considered that the action of the blade might provide a range of information at different points in the mark as a result of incision and subsequent removal of the weapon. For this reason, it was proposed the kerf should be deliberately scored in three sections: the main channel, and the two mark tips (Fig. 3). The mark tips are the defined extremities of the kerf, and named according to their proximity to the nearest anatomical border e.g. the anterior tip is the end of the kerf approaching the anterior border of the bone. Note the very different shapes of the tips in Figure 3; the anterior tip narrowly tapers, in contrast to the flared and rounded posterior tip.

The main channel is body of the kerf, located between the anterior and posterior tips.

Features evaluated during the creation of the recording sheets include:
- Dimensional data (width, depth, length, etc.)
- Recording visible striae
- Recording the edge or 'margin' morphology of the kerf
- Cross-sectional shape
- Floor data, including definition and overall shape
- Other observable characteristics

Table 1 highlights the variation in kerf features examined or observed across a number of disciplines. Loe and Cox (2005:12) currently detail the most comprehensive range of characteristics; however, these refer to striations on bone that do not necessarily describe incision marks specifically. The striation, or kerf, characteristics may also be used to describe chopping and scraping marks on the surface of bone. The use of the term "striation" in this context is not to be confused with the internal striations inherent within a mark as the result of the cutting action of the tool against a hard surface (Burd and Greene, 1948), again illustrating how disparity in terminology across subject areas exists.

Kerf characteristics were defined, and scored accordingly. In addition to the criteria listed, supplementary notes were taken to catalogue any additional observations or findings for later evaluation and analysis. Details of terms and definitions are listed below:

Tip-specific characteristics

Shape
The overall marginal shape of the each tip was noted. Several different shapes were observed (Fig. 4), including square, rounded, tapered, bulbous and flared or open ended tips.

Bifurcation
In some circumstances, the tip was observed to 'fork', or split in two directions (Fig. 5).

Wall and profile characteristics

Cross-section
The overall profile shape of the kerf exhibited shapes including V, U, |_|, W, and a number of variations in-between. The cross-sectional shape is influenced by the gradient of the walls, and the overall shape and definition of the floor.

Wall gradient
The gradient is the level of slope that can be attributed to each kerf wall. The anatomical prefix (vertebral/sternal) denotes the rib end to which the wall is closest. A very steep gradient exhibits approximately a 90° angle with the kerf floor.

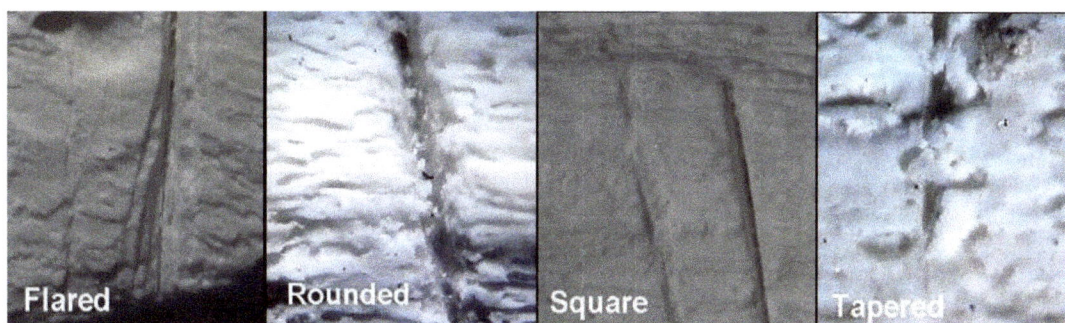

Figure 4. Showing typical variations of tip shape, at magnifications of 180x to 525x on the Projectina Comparison Macroscope.

Wall projections
Wall projections are bony protrusions, distinguished from other bony debris because the projections are attached to the kerf wall (Fig. 6).

Margin characteristics

Margins
The margins can be defined as the surface boundaries of the kerf, or the edges of the cut. Each margin is scored separately and can be identified by use of an anatomical prefix to denote directional proximity (in this case, sternal or vertebral). Two separate characteristics were scored for the kerf margins; regularity and definition.

Margin regularity
Regularity refers to the linear nature of the margins; continuous deviation from a linear form can be categorised as an irregular margin.

Margin definition
Kerf margin definition is scored according to the sharpness, clarity and precision of the edge. In Figure 7, mark 11 exhibits two well regular, defined edges, whereas mark 12 exhibits a defined vertebral margin and an undefined but regular sternal margin.

Margin splitting
Observation of the presence or absence of cracking at the kerf margins was also undertaken. Margin splitting was not observed commonly in current experimental samples, but was observed in preliminary test cuts made by the author. This may have been an result of harsher preliminary preparation techniques with a much longer maceration period, which also involved continuous use of enzyme detergent.

Lateral ridging
This is a characteristic 'peaking' at either or both margins, with a ridge forming along the margin's edge (Fig. 8). Alunni-Perret *et al.* (2005:780) documented a similar phenomenon known as "unilateral raising", as it was observed at only one margin.

Lateral ridging location
In the experimental sample, when the presence of lateral ridging was noted, its location at either or both margins was also observed, and labelled according to the margin's relative anatomical position (vertebral or sternal).

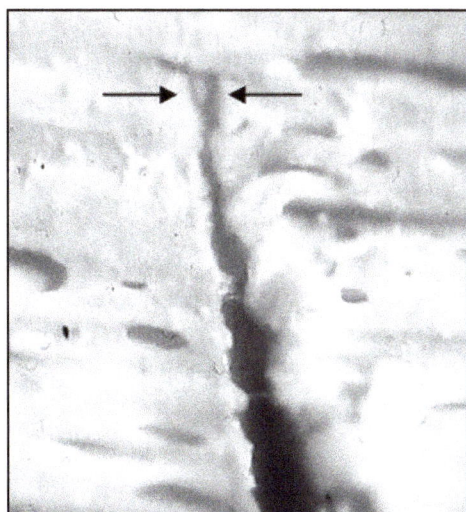

Figure 5. Serrated blade cut anterior tip exhibiting bifurcation (superior surface) at 525x on Projectina Comparison Macroscope.

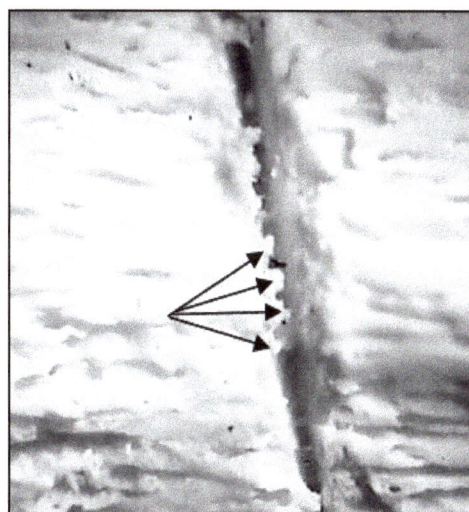

Figure 6. Serrated blade cut displaying wall projections (shown by the arrows) to vertebral margin at 300x magnification.

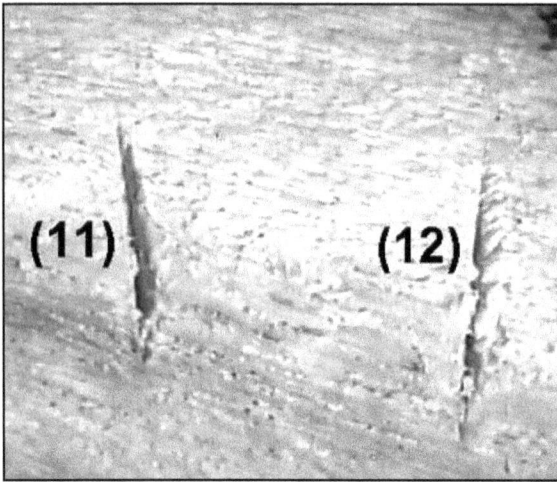

Figure 7. Serrated Blade, marks 11 and 12 at 105x magnification on a Projectina Comparison Macroscope.

Floor characteristics

Kerf floor

This can be defined as the nadir of the kerf; the area connecting the kerf walls. Observation of floor characteristics can be problematic, depending on both cross-section shape and the width of the mark, which can sometimes be too narrow for observations to be made. The presence of wall projections and debris in the kerf can also prevent a full examination of the floor by obscuring it from view. The characteristics scored for the kerf floor include definition, splitting, and arbitrary width.

Floor definition

Definition scores the precision and clarity of the floor shape, and in particular the relationship of the morphology at which the floor and the walls join. Clear boundaries between the floor and walls show a defined relationship, and any ambiguity in this relationship is scored as an undefined floor.

Floor width

The floor width is the arbitrary total width of the kerf floor, from wall to wall.

Floor splitting

The presence of observable cracks in the kerf floor (shown in Fig. 9) is known as floor splitting.

Debris

Debris within the mark varied in size, shape and composition. The presence of debris inhibited the observation of some marks, but in each case was catalogued according to the following criteria:

Crushing

Debris in the kerf that has a granular appearance.

Flaking

Debris in the kerf that has a flat, thin appearance.

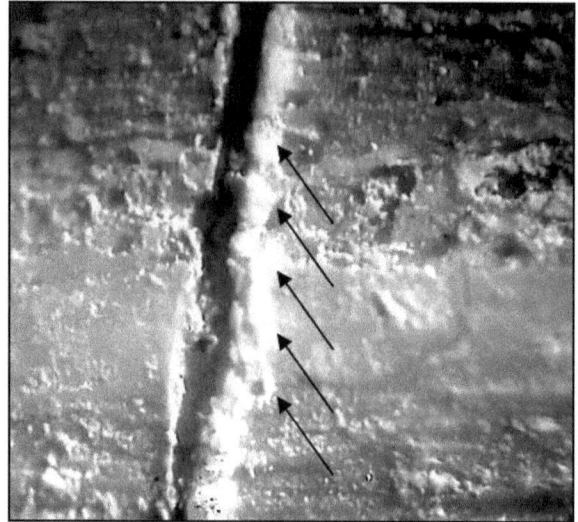

Figure 8. Serrated main channel imaged on a Projectina Comparison Macroscope at 300x. Sternal is left. Note the presence of lateral ridging, particularly on the vertebral margin of the kerf.

Large

Large fragments included those that were 0.5mm or larger in diameter, length or breadth at a magnification of 40x.

Fine

Small fragments included those that were less than 0.5mm in diameter, length or breadth at a magnification of 40x.

Debris type

Kerf debris was categorised into three observable types; bone, tissue and metal.

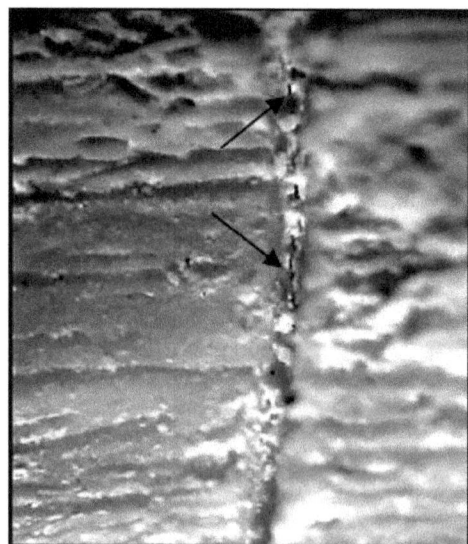

Figure 9. Serrated cut at 300x magnification. The arrows indicate the location of splitting in the floor of the kerf.

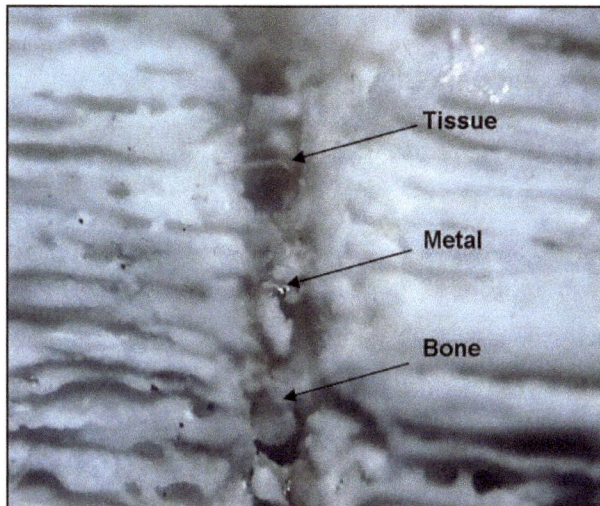

Figure 10. Fine cut kerf with all three debris types observable within, and a textured surrounding surface. Magnification: 525x.

Bone surface characteristics

Bone porosity
The presence of surface pores in the surrounding bone was noted. The presence of multiple pores in numerous areas surrounding the mark is classified as a porous surface. Figure 10 exhibits a porous bone surface.

Bone texture
The surface of bone was scored according to its appearance. Cortical bone that showed little surface topography was classed as smooth, whereas a visibly undulating appearance was classified as textured (as can be seen in Fig. 10). In areas of mixed topography, classification focussed around the immediate area of the incision for scoring purposes.

Bone gradient
The bone gradient is the degree of surface slope of the area surrounding the cut. A level surface was categorised with no gradient, a surface with a slope apparently greater than $45°$ was classified as a steep gradient, and a surface with an angle less than $45°$ was a shallow gradient.

Analysis

All data were transcribed to numeric values, to allow statistical analysis using the SPSS 13.0 package. The chi-square test for independence was used for analysis, in conjunction with the Fisher's exact test, where appropriate. Three sets of variables were tested, including cut mark characteristics, knife characteristics and bone characteristics.

Results

Bone surface characteristics

In making basic observations about the bone surface surrounding each mark according to porosity, texture and gradient, the chi-square test indicates that these particular characteristics are not significantly influential ($p =\leq 0.05$) on any of the cut mark features.

As incisions were carried out on both the superior and inferior surfaces of the bone, this was tested as a possible source of influence on cut mark characteristics themselves (Table 3). When tested against blade type, the cut mark surface does have a significant relationship with main channel (MC) floor definition ($p=0.036$). No significant results are recorded with the anterior or posterior tips of serrated blades. For scalloped blades, no significant results are recorded for the main channel or the tips. Fine-edged blades show relationships between surface and anterior tip (AT) bifurcation ($p=0.000$), and lateral ridging ($p=0.025$).

No significant results exist for the posterior tip (PT), but the main channel of fine blade cuts exhibits a relationship between surface and depth consistency of the mark ($\chi^2 = 6.348$, $p =0.042$, df = 2). When the marks are examined as a complete group (n.=250), the anterior tip provides most significant results, in relation to bifurcation ($p=0.000$), lateral ridging ($p=0.032$), and lateral ridging location ($p=0.002$). The main channel also indicates relationships between projection size ($p=0.027$) and lateral ridging location ($p=0.000$).

Blade and knife characteristics

Cutting edge
The cutting edge of each knife was classified as either a single or a double sided blade, depending on whether the blade had been ground, or sharpened, on one or both sides of the cutting edge. There are several significant relationships to report for both tips and the main channel. The cutting edge shows significant relationships between floor definition ($p=0.042$), floor splitting ($p=0.017$) and flaking debris ($p=0.003$) for the anterior tip. For details of significant characteristics for the tips and main channel, see Tables 4 and 5.

Blade type
The blades used have three categories; serrated, scalloped, and fine types. For details of significant characteristics, see Table 6.

Blade use
Analysis revealed no significant data relating to mark characteristics and blade use or blade wear.

Knife type
For details of knife types used, see Table 1. Table 7 shows the results and surprisingly, only one main channel characteristic has a significant relationship with knife type; that of depth consistency ($p=0.000$). Knife type

Table 3. Values for kerf characteristics and their relationship with the bone surface (superior/inferior).

Kerf Characteristics	Location in kerf	X^2	Degrees of freedom	Significance $p =$	N=
Bifurcation	AT	18.120	2	0.000	250
Crushing debris	AT	8.041	2	0.018	248
Lateral Ridging (LR)	AT	6.854	2	0.032	248
LR Location	AT	17.289	4	0.002	245
	MC	23.725	10	0.000	237
Projection Size	MC	10.995	4	0.027	247

Table 4. Values for tip characteristics of the kerf and their relationship with the blade cutting edge.

Kerf Characteristics	Location in kerf	X^2	Degrees of freedom	Significance $p =$	N=
Floor definition	AT	6.347	2	0.042	247
	PT	11.947	2	0.003	245
Floor splitting	AT	8.161	2	0.017	247
	PT	13.447	2	0.001	249
Flaking debris	AT	11.854	2	0.003	249
	PT	12.051	2	0.001	249
Tip shape	PT	14.677	4	0.005	250
X-section	PT	10.951	3	0.012	250
Vertebral gradient	PT	17.612	5	0.003	250
No. projections	PT	11.129	3	0.011	250
Overall margin definition	PT	6.940	2	0.031	247

Table 5. Values for main channel characteristics of the kerf and their relationship with the blade cutting edge.

Kerf Charcteristics	Location in kerf	X^2	Degrees of freedom	Significance $p =$	N=
Depth	MC	16.913	3	0.001	248
Depth consistency	MC	8.192	2	0.017	240
No. projections	MC	8.334	3	0.040	247
Projection size	MC	10.084	4	0.039	247
Overall margin definition	MC	12.350	2	0.002	243
Crushing debris	MC	25.991	2	0.000	247
Lateral ridging (LR)	MC	12.864	2	0.002	242
LR Location	MC	18.980	4	0.001	237

shows significant relationships with both the anterior and posterior tip. The anterior tip is significant for both cross-section ($p=0.002$) and floor definition ($p=0.000$), whereas only floor definition is significant for the posterior tip ($p=0.000$).

Discussion

Morphological characteristics of the bone surface were observed in this experiment, and had no significant effect on cut mark kerf characteristics. Although bone surface features do not influence marks, the anatomical surface on which the mark is made does indicate a relationship; this could be an artefact of manual application of the knives to bone, and therefore it may be valuable to carry out comparisons of manual marks and machine-made cuts.

Examining the mark in discrete sections rather than making general observations of the overall kerf proved valuable; from the experimental data, detailed examination of the tips of a cut can provide almost as much information as the main channel. Whilst there are some characteristics that exhibit consistently significant relationships with a number of different knife features, there are some features that show relationships with different areas of the kerf, e.g. floor splitting is related to the cutting edge type for the tips of the kerf, but not the main channel. This may also be a result of the manual application of the knife, as subtle variations in the

Table 6. Values for kerf characteristics and their relationship with blade type.

Kerf Characteristics	Location in kerf	χ2	Degrees of freedom	Significance p =	N=
Consistent depth	MC	24.474	4	**0.000**	240
No. projections	MC	32.839	6	**0.000**	247
Projection size	MC	23.163	8	**0.003**	247
Floor splitting	MC	11.563	4	**0.021**	248
X-section	MC	17.982	6	**0.006**	246
	PT	16.658	6	**0.011**	250
Floor definition	MC	11.880	4	**0.018**	242
	PT	21.023	4	**0.000**	245
	AT	16.330	4	**0.003**	247
Bifurcation	AT	7.397	2	**0.025**	250
Flaking debris	AT	22.894	4	**0.000**	247

Table 7. Values for kerf characteristics and their relationship with knife type.

Kerf Characteristics	Location in kerf	χ2	Degrees of freedom	Significance p =	N=
Depth consistency (All blades)	MC	67.251	10	**0.000**	240
X-Section (All blades)	AT	35.524	15	**0.002**	250
Floor definition (All blades)	AT	33.173	10	**0.000**	247
	PT	35.160	10	**0.000**	245
Floor definition (Fine Blades)	AT	16.679	6	**0.010**	159
	PT	12.991	6	**0.043**	158
X-Section (Fine Blades)	AT	26.237	9	**0.002**	160

positioning and angle of the knife may result in different parts of the blade having more or less contact with the bone surface. Lifting the knife blade slightly as the knife is withdrawn from the bone may mean that features are more clearly recorded in some areas of the kerf and not others; for example, the presence of cross-section relationships for the main channel and posterior tip, but not the anterior tip. It is interesting to note that common features used for identification and discrimination purposes, such as cross-sectional shape, are not as prominent in the results as might be expected. Instead, wall features like projections, and characteristics of the kerf floor feature predominantly across the variables studied. Floor definition is the most prevalent, showing significant relationships in 46% of the knife variables tested. Lateral ridging, documented by Alunni-Perret *et al.* (2005) as unilateral raising, is also a significant characteristic in this sample of knives, and it has now been observed here in manually-applied cuts as well as machine cuts. The 'raising' or ridging has now also been observed bilaterally; a feature not documented in Alunni-Perret *et al.* (2005). Lateral ridging is a result of the blade entering the bone at an angle other than 90° (Alunni-Perret *et al.*, 2005). The fact that the ridging occurs bilaterally in the current sample may be a result of tilting the knife during the incision and withdrawal of the blade.

Debris is also present as a significant feature, however the preparation process may have had an influence on the debris observed. It may be possible to examine a range of techniques, including ultrasonication, and maceration without the addition of heat or biological or chemical agents, and observe knife cuts made by the same weapon to determine how significantly the preparation techniques affect debris within the cut. If the size and type of debris can be established as functional features in cut mark analysis, the marks should be examined before cleaning in order to record the type and relative frequency of debris in the cut. Common practice of cleaning the cuts before examination may therefore be removing discriminating and useful information.

The lack of significant information from the blade use analysis does not necessarily preclude it as a relevant variable. The sample of used knives was small (n=2), so further work needs to be carried out to investigate this effect. It should also be noted that the knives documented as "used" had been used only in preliminary experiments, and level of usage was light. Further experiments may involve knives with records of heavy usage or deliberate damage to the blade.

Further work in this area will involve the direct comparison of experimental marks made by machine or by manual application, as well as expanding the existing sample of knives, in particular with more examples of scalloped and serrated blades. The experimental marks examined were still fresh, and consideration should be given to the fact that in bone preservation may affect the survival of microscopic features (Smith *et al.*, 2007), and this effect has not yet been fully explored. Shipman and Rose (1983) examined the affects of sedimentary abrasion and all diagnostic, microscopic features of cut marks were obliterated in a five- hour period of geological tumbling (approximately equivalent to a distance travelled of 3.6km). They acknowledge that sedimentary impact was more continuous, and the velocity more constant than likely to be realistic, but it does demonstrate that extraneous factors may have an effect on the cut marks, and therefore subsequent analysis. Bromage and Boyde (1984) observed that the use of enzyme detergent in preparation techniques removed striae from the cuts; no research has been conducted into enzymatic decomposition and its effect on cut-marks in bone. Other taphonomic variables, such as burial environment, immersion in water, and weathering may have an affect on kerf characteristics but have not yet been investigated. The need to record cut mark data consistently and accurately should continue to be addressed, with re-evaluation of existing criteria, based on greater experience of cut mark observation and analysis.

Conclusions

Microscopic analysis of incision marks on bone is not a new concept; but published data in a forensic context is still novel. The broad spectrum of knowledge supplied by other disciplines gives a strong foundation from which to learn and progress. By examining some of the features used in the analysis of cut marks in archaeology and palaeoanthropology, a number of these characteristics are suggested to be informative for metal cut marks, in addition to their existing use for stone and bone tools. Relationships have been established between blade characteristics and kerf features including; kerf depth consistency; the number of wall projections and their relative sizes; floor definition and floor splitting; cross-sectional shape; debris type, and lateral ridging and its location. The extents of these relationships are yet to be established, and their success as tools for forensic analysis needs to be explored further. Existing literature should be challenged by rigorous testing and re-evaluation of methods, and every effort should be made to approach consistency and accuracy in both the observation and subsequent documentation of cut marks on bone.

Acknowledgements

Many thanks to Tal Simmons for her support and feedback. The assistance of Eddie Taylor and Tony Morton-Jones with statistical analysis was invaluable, and grateful thanks go to Sal Tracey for her technical assistance in the laboratory, and also Rachel Adlam and Adam Wilcox for their consultation and support.

Literature Cited

Adelson, L. 1974. *The Pathology of Homicide. A Vade Mecum for Pathologist, Prosecutor and Defence Counsel.* Springfield, Illinois: Charles C Thomas.

Alunni-Perret, V., Muller-Bolla, M., Laugier, J.P., Lupi-Pegurier, L., Bertrand, M. F., Staccini, P., Bolla, M. and Quatrehomme, G. 2005. "Scanning Electron Microscopy Analysis of Experimental Bone Hacking Trauma". *Journal of Forensic Sciences*, 50: 796-801.

Bartelink, E.J., Wiersema, J.M., and Demaree, R.S. 2001. "Quantitative Analysis of Sharp Force Trauma: An Application of Scanning Electron Microscopy in Forensic Anthropology." *Journal of Forensic Sciences* 46: 1288-1293.

Blumenschine, R.J., Marean, C.W., and Capaldo, S.D. 1996. "Blind Tests of Inter-analyst Correspondence and Accuracy in the Identification of Cut Marks, Percussion Marks, and Carnivore Tooth Marks on Bone Surfaces." *Journal of Archaeological Science* 23: 493-507.

Bromage, T.G., and Boyde, A. 1984. "Microscopic Criteria for the Determination of Directionality of Cutmarks on Bone". *American Journal of Physical Anthropology* 65: 359-366.

Bunn, H.T. 1981. "Archaeological Evidence for Meat-Eating by Plio-Pleistocene Hominids from Koobi Fora and Olduvai Gorge." *Nature* 291: 574-577.

Burd, D.Q. and Greene, R.S. 1948. "Tool Mark Comparisons in Criminal Cases." *Journal of Criminal Law and Criminology* 39: 379-391.

Chadwick, E.K.J., Nicol, A.C., Lane, J.V. and Gray, T.G.F. 1999. "Biomechanics of Knife Stab Attacks." *Forensic Science International* 105: 35-44.

Coleman, K., Hird, C., and Povey, D. 2006. *Violent Crime Overview: Homicide and Gun Crime. Supplementary Volume to Crime in England and Wales 2004/2005.* London: Home Office Statistical Bulletin. 49.

DiMaio, D.J. and DiMaio, V.J.M. 1993. *Forensic Pathology.* Boca Raton: CRC Press.

Eickhoff, S. and Herrmann, B. 1985. "Surface Marks on Bone from a Neolithic Collective Grave (Odagsen, Lower Saxony). A Study on Differential Diagnosis." *Journal of Human Evolution* 14:163-274.

Fenton, T.W., Birkby, W.H., and Cornelison, J. 2003. "A Fast and Safe Non-Bleaching Method for Forensic Skeletal Preparation." *Journal of Forensic Sciences* 48: 274-276.

Greenfield, H.J. 1999. "The Origins of Metallurgy: Distinguishing Stone from Metal Cut-marks on Bones from Archaeological Sites." *Journal of Archaeological Science* 26: 797-808.

Houck, M.M. 1998. "Skeletal Trauma and the Individualization of Knife Marks in Bones". In Reichs, K. J. (ed.) *Forensic Osteology: Advances in the Identification of Human Remains."* Springfield, Illinois: Charles C. Thomas. 410-425.

Hunt, A.C., and Cowling, R.J. 1991. "Murder by Stabbing." *Forensic Science International* 52: 107-112.

Knight, B. 1975 "The Dynamics of Stab Wounds." *Forensic Science* 6: 249-255.

Loe, L. and Cox, M. 2005. "Peri- and post mortem surface features on archaeological human bone: why they should not be ignored and a protocol for their identification and interpretation." In Zakrzewski, S.R. and Clegg, M. (eds.) *Proceedings of the Fifth Annual Conference of the British Association for Biological Anthropology and Osteoarchaeology*. Oxford: BAR Publishing. 11-21.

O'Callaghan, P.T., Jones, M.D., James, D.S., Leadbeatter, S., Holt, C.A., and Nokes, L.D.M. 1999. "Dynamics of Stab Wounds: Force Required for Penetration of Various Cadaveric Tissues." *Forensic Science International* 104: 173-178.

Olsen, S. L. 1988. "The Identification of Stone and Metal Tool Marks on Bone Artefacts." In Olsen, S.L., (ed.) *Scanning Electron Microscopy in Archaeology.* British Archaeological Reports, International Series 452. Oxford: BAR Publishing. 337-363.

Olsen, S.L., and Shipman, P. 1988. Surface Modification on Bone: Trampling versus Butchery. *Journal of Archaeological Science* 15: 535-553.

Potts, R., and Shipman, P. 1981. "Cutmarks Made by Stone Tools on Bones from Olduvai Gorge, Tanzania." *Nature* 291: 577-580.

Prieto, J. 2007. "Stab Wounds: The Contribution of Forensic Anthropology: A Case Study". In Brickley, M. and Ferllini R. (eds.) *Forensic Anthropology: Case Studies from Europe.* Springfield, Illinois: Charles C. Thomas. 19-37.

Rao, V.J. and Hart, R. 1983. "Tool Mark Determination in Cartilage of Stabbing Victims" *Journal of Forensic Sciences* 28: 794-799.

Rogde, S., Hougen, H.P. and Poulsen, K. 2000. "Homicide by Sharp Force in Two Scandinavian Capitals." *Forensic Science International* 109: 135-145.

Rouse, D.A. 1994. "Patterns of Stab Wounds: A Six Year Study." *Medicine, Science and the Law* 34: 67-71.

Rose, J. 1983. "A Replication Technique for Scanning Electron Microscopy." *American Journal of Physical Anthropology* 62: 255-261.

Saferstein, R. 2001. *Criminalistics: An Introduction to Forensic Science.* Seventh Edition. New Jersey: Prentice Hall.

Schmidt, U., and Pollak, S. 2006. "Sharp Force Injuries in Clinical Forensic Medicine: Findings in Victims and Perpetrators." *Forensic Science International* 159: 113-118.

Shipman, P. 1981. "Applications of Scanning Electron Microscopy to Taphonomic Problems." In: Cantwell, A.M., Griffen, J.B. and Rothschild, (eds.) *The Research Potential of Anthropological Museum Collections.* Annals of the New York Academy of Science 376: 357-385.

Shipman, P. 1983. "Early Hominid Lifestyle: Hunting and Gathering or Foraging and Scavenging?" *British Archaeological Report* 163: 31-49.

Shipman, P. and Rose, J. 1983. "Early Hominid Hunting, Butchering, and Carcass-Processing Behaviours: Approaches to the Fossil Record." *Journal of Anthropological Archaeology* 2: 57-96.

Shipman, P. and Rose, J. 1988. "Bone Tools: An Experimental Approach." *Scanning Electron Microscopy in Archaeology.* British Archaeological Reports, International Series 452. Oxford: BAR Publishing. 303-333.

Smith, M.J., and Brickley, M.B. 2004. "Analysis and Interpretation of Flint Toolmarks found on Bones from West Tump Long Barrow, Gloucestershire." *International Journal of Osteoarchaeology* 14: 18-33.

Smith, M.J. Brickley, M.B., and Leach, S.L. 2007. "Experimental Evidence for Lithic Projectile Injuries: Improving Identification of an Under-recognised Phenomenon." *Journal of Archaeological Science* 34: 540-553.

Spitz, W.U. 1993. "Sharp Force Injury." In Spitz, W.U. (ed.) *Spitz and Fisher's Medicolegal Investigation of Death: Guidelines for the Application of Pathology to Crime Investigation.* Springfield, Illinois: Charles, C. Thomas. 252-309.

Symes, S.A .1992. *Morphology of Saw Marks in Human Bone: Identification of Class Characteristics.* Ph.D. thesis, University of Tennessee.

Symes, S.A., Williams, J.A., Murray, E.A., Hoffman, J.M., Holland, T.D., Saul, J.M., Saul, F.P. and Pope, E.J. 2002. "Taphonomic Context of Sharp-Trauma in Suspected Cases of Human Mutilation and Dismemberment." In Haglund, W.D. and Sorg, S.M.H.

(eds.) *Advances in Forensic Taphonomy*. Boca Raton: CRC Press. 403-434.

Tucker, B.K., Hutchison, D.L., Gilliland, M.F.G., Charles, T.M., Daniel, H.J. and Wolfe, L.D. 2001. "Microscopic Characteristics of Hacking Trauma." *Journal of Forensic Sciences* 46: 234-240.

Wenham, S.J. 1989. "Anatomical Interpretations of Anglo-Saxon England" In: Chadwic-Hawkes, S. (ed.) *Weapons and Warfare in Anglo-Saxon England.* Oxford: Oxford University Committee for Archaeology.123-139.

"All the outward tinsel which distinguishes man from man will have then vanished..."*. an assessment of the value of post-medieval human remains to migration studies

Garret "Irish in London" cited by J Garwood (1853: 316)

Natasha Powers

Museum of London Archaeology Service (MoLAS), Mortimer Wheeler House
46 Eagle Wharf Road, London, N1 7ED
e-mail address for correspondence: npowers@museumoflondon.org.uk

Abstract

The research value of post-medieval assemblages has been recognised only recently. Whilst such assemblages have been used to test osteological methods, there has been no systematic examination of evidence for population movement. Proposed artefactual, funerary, epigraphic and osteological indicators of migration were evaluated for a post-medieval assemblage, to determine whether culturally specific population differences were present and if so, whether interpretation would be possible in a framework devoid of supporting documentary evidence. Assessment data for a group of 747 Catholics interred in East London during the mid-nineteenth century were chosen, as historic evidence suggested many of this group had migrated from Ireland during the potato famine.

The results demonstrated the problems of interpreting cemetery assemblages. Epigraphic evidence proved to be the only credible indicator of migration. No differences in burial practices were identified. Grave inclusions and furniture appeared more culturally specific. Probable patterns were present in the osteological data, but interpretation proved highly problematic. The adult sex ratio was similar to contemporary sites, providing no clear indications of economic migration. Lower than expected rates of non-specific and some specific infections, sub-adult enamel hypoplasia and trauma suggested that the 'osteological paradox' could be a significant factor.

Isotopic analyses may be the only dependable indicator of migration for ancient remains. It is argued that well-documented post-medieval burials, such as this group, would make ideal test cases for the analyses of isotopes as indicators of geographic mobility, to determine whether apparent differences can be correlated with known migration events.

Keywords: Post-medieval, migration, famine, isotopes, London, stress

Introduction

In 2002, the Research Framework for Greater London Archaeology (Nixon *et al.,* 2002), identified the examination of cultural groups as a primary theme for the post-medieval period. However, the contribution of the study of human remains to this end and the potential of these remains to provide data for migration studies has not been widely recognised. Skeletal material, for which historic records survive, provides test cases for theoretical discussion of cultural identifiers in the archaeological record. This paper examines suggested indicators of cultural difference which could be used to identify migrant groups, with reference to an unusual post-medieval sample excavated by the Museum of London Archaeology Service during 2005. The osteological and archaeological data presented here resulted from assessment level observations, not full skeletal analysis, and should be considered only an initial indicator of the full potential of the assemblage. Results are open to alteration following full analysis.

London and migration

The economic opportunities afforded by the Capital have long made London a focus for migration. In 1847-48,

famine in Ireland initiated mass migration to England. This was encouraged by cheap travel on the new steamboats and the possibility of achieving higher wages than those available at home. In 1851 alone, 257,372 people left Ireland, the Irish in London outnumbering those in Belfast during this period (Garwood, 1853: 300, 245). By 1897, an estimated 24% of the population of Whitechapel were immigrants (Sherwell, 1897).

The cemetery sample

The cemetery of the Catholic Mission of St. Mary and St. Michael, Commercial Road, Whitechapel in the East End of London was in use for a period of just eleven years. The church served a congregation composed predominantly of poor Irish labourers (Murphy, 1991). In 1842, a building plot was purchased and subdivided to provide a burial ground. Although construction of the church did not begin until 1853, the cemetery was consecrated on 24 July 1843. Burials continued until the site was closed on 1 May 1854. An area of the cemetery later became part of the Bishop Challoner Primary School playground (Miles and Powers, 2006).

During 2005, in advance of development for a new school building, archaeological excavation of a large

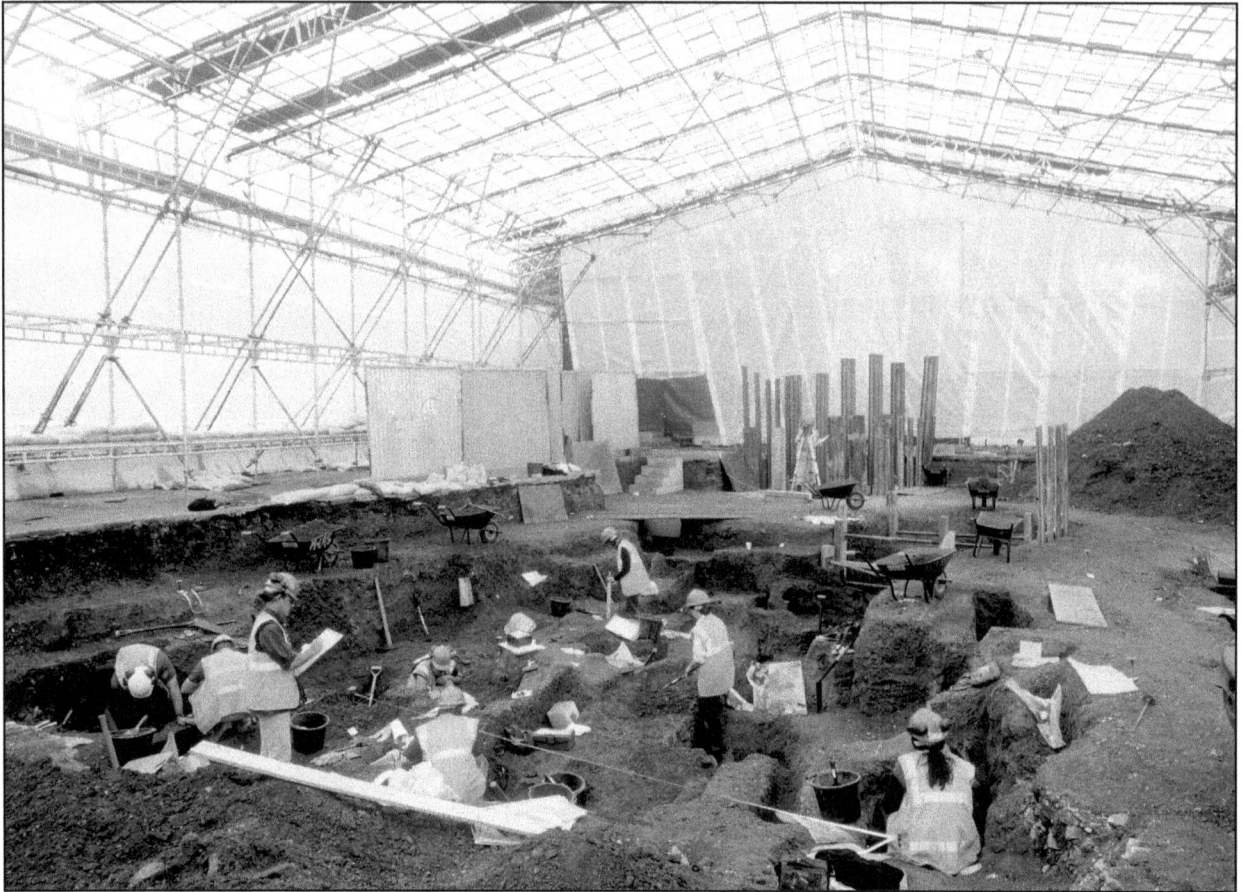

Figure 1. Excavation in progress at St. Mary and St. Michael's ©MoLAS.

portion of the burial ground revealed stacked wooden coffins, in the order of eight individuals interred within each deeply cut grave, and no intercutting of the graves (Fig.1). Partially legible coffin plates were recovered from 194 contexts, roughly one quarter of the total number of burials recovered. Osteological assessment, indicated that there were a total of 747 individuals: 293 adults (39%), 454 sub-adults (61%) (Miles and Powers, 2006).

With the historic characterisation of Whitechapel, and the nature of the cemetery in mind, attempts were made to establish and quantify the presence of recent incomers within the buried population at St. Mary and St. Michael's and to investigate the possibility of identifying known, historic migration events amongst skeletal samples.

Evidence for immigrant populations

The written word: epigraphic evidence

Of the 49 individuals for whom surname could be confidently established, 32 names were determined to be of probable Irish origin (65%) by comparison with on-line genealogical databases (www.censusfinder.com). One Italian and a probable Portuguese individual were also present (Table 1). The epigraphic data is therefore heavily suggestive of a migrant group. Though comparison with London parish cemeteries of similar date would undoubtedly also reveal individuals with

many of these names, the high proportion seen here, coupled with the religious information and the results of the ongoing historic research, supports the theory that the cemetery population was largely of Irish origin.

Surname evidence alone cannot determine whether the individuals buried at St. Mary and St. Michael's, or their forebears, originated beyond England. Nor can it disentangle the complicated relationship between ethnic or cultural origin and one's own perception of cultural identity. Expatriate communities may feel strong cultural ties to their country of origin for many generations after an initial migration event. Contemporary documents make it clear that in the 1840s, established Irish 'Cockneys' were unhappy at the new wave of migration which occurred as the result of the famine (Garwood, 1853). This indicates that Irish families, and thus Irish surnames, had been resident in the East End for many years. Since surnames are passed through the male line, epigraphic data is less useful when examining the female population: a non-local surname may simply indicate a 'native' Londoner who had married into an Irish family.

The way in which Garwood and other writers of the time discuss immigrants suggests that the Irish of the 1850s formed a fairly discreet, even insular community: it was estimated at this time that one third of those living in the Commercial Road parish spoke the Irish language almost exclusively (McDonnell, 1969: 434). The linguistic issues were so great that the Archbishop of Westminster was petitioned for an Irish speaking Priest to minister more

Table 1. Surnames of non-English origin amongst the St. Mary and St. Micheal's cemetery population.

Surname	Christian name	Title	Surname origin	Suggested or alternative spelling?
Alphonso	-	-	Italian?	-
Boland	Ambrose	Master	Irish	modern version of O' Bolan
Broschan	John	Master	Irish?	Brosnan
Coakly	Cornelus	Master	Irish	-
Creagie	..e..en	-	Irish?	Cregan
Cullin?	Catherine	-	Irish	Quinlan
D..no..y	Mary Jane	-	Irish	Donolly?
Dono..n	...rn	Mr	Irish	-
Dowd.	Thomas?	-	Irish?	-
Driscoll	C....	Master	Irish	-
Fealy	-	-	Irish	Feeley
Ha...gton	Thomas	Master	Irish	Haughton
Hogen	Daniel	Master	Irish	Hogan
K...dy	Margaret Eup..	-	Irish?	Kenedy
Lineha..	Ann	-	Irish	-
Lyons	Mary	Miss	Irish?	-
Magreen?	Christopher	Master	Irish?	-
Mahoney	Michael	-	Irish	-
Mahoney	E...	Miss	Irish	-
Mahoney	-	Miss	Irish	-
McDer..mt	Marga..	-	Irish	-
McN..lly	..iget	-	Irish	-
Muldavy	Bridgett	-	Irish	-
Murphy	..len	Miss	Irish	-
Murray	Annora	-	Irish?	-
Niele	..organa Sara..	-	Irish	Neely
Penethera	Miguel	Mr	Portuguese?	-
Rega..	William Robert	Master	Irish	Regan
Regan	John	Mr	Irish	-
Rigan..	-	-	Irish?	may be spelling of Regan
Ryan	Michael	Mr	Irish	-
S..livan	P..	Mr	Irish	Sullivan
Sul...	-	-	Irish	Sullivan
Sullivan	Timothy	-	Irish	Sullivan

effectively to the local population (Westminster Diocesan Archive, R/74, letter dated 5 Dec 1853). Despite this, it would be unwise to assume that no culturally mixed marriages took place.

Demography

It has been suggested that demographic patterns can identify populations containing large groups of economic migrants, as these are predominantly younger males. An examination of records of a west Chicago poor house from 1851-1869 indicated most of the inmates were Irish migrants and showed that males made up the largest portion of the population (Grauer *et al.*, 1998). However, whether the poor house can be taken as a good proxy for the entire migrant population is debatable. Unfortunately, no records exist pertaining directly to the living

population served by the cemetery of St. Mary and St. Michael, but further documentary research during full analysis may bring to light records pertaining to the wider area of the East End against which the cemetery population can be compared.

The assessment data for the St. Mary and St. Michael assemblage resulted in an adult sex ratio of 1.4: 1 (149 male, 109 female). In most populations, the sex ratio at birth is 106 males to 100 females (Rousham, 1999: 37; Rousham and Humphrey, 2002: 128). The adult sex ratio in any population will be affected by many environmental and genetic factors. Rousham and Humphrey (2002: 137) state that "poverty, social disadvantage and disease are strong selective agents in both contemporary and historical populations...[which]...may shape the genetic and demographic structure of the population". Male infant mortality rates are generally higher than those of females (Pollard and Hyatt, 1999: 2), with male infants more susceptible to respiratory problems and infectious disease (Rousham, 1999: 38). Such factors would be expected to result in a levelling of the sex ratio into adulthood (*ibid.*).

Archaeological samples frequently show a slight male bias in the adult population which has been suggested to be the result of methodological issues (Walker, 1995). Notwithstanding this point, the adult sex ratio at St. Mary and St. Michael's is similar to numerous contemporary London sites (Fig. 2). For example, at St. Marylebone a sex ratio of 1.2:1 was noted (105 males, 86 females) (Miles and Powers, 2006), whilst a ratio of 1.3:1 was seen at St. Luke's Old Street (Boyle *et al.*, 2005: 187). As such it is difficult to conclude that the slightly raised proportion of males at this site is the result of the migration of a predominantly male group from Ireland. Whilst it could be argued that the economic migration of males was a significant factor throughout London at this time, and so an increased male representation would be present in all cemetery groups from the city, the demographic structure seen at St. Mary and St. Michael's does not appear to reflect an unusual or dramatic influx of males. It is interesting to note that England was also said to provide refuge for young Catholic women who had 'fallen from virtue' (Garwood, 1853: 305). Perhaps this led to a more even sex distribution than anticipated? It is also possible that there was little overall population bias in the migrant group. Writing in 1855, Watts Philips talked of entire families, men women and children migrating to London as a group (Jackson, 2006: 128). Full osteological analysis, which includes a more detailed estimate of adult age at death, will enable the interpretation to be refined taking into account varying sex ratios across the age groups.

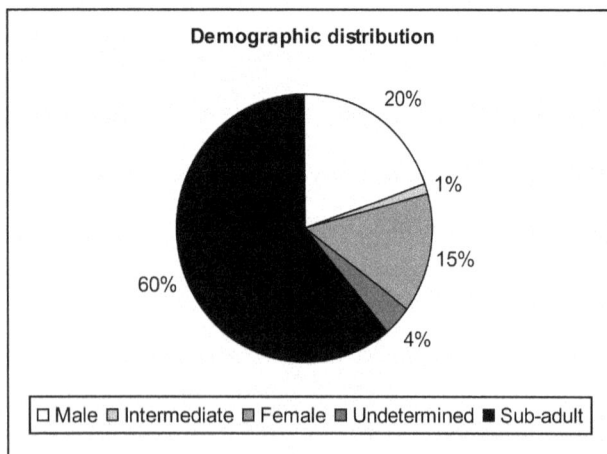

Figure 2. Demographic distribution of the buried population from St. Mary and St. Michael's (assessment level data).

Archaeological and artefactual evidence: funerary practices

One possible cultural distinction could be the manner, orientation and location of a grave. The diversity of post-medieval burial practices has been stressed by past authors (Roberts and Cox, 2003). Within burial grounds practical use of space dictated uniformity in the positioning and alignment of graves, and pragmatism often dictated burial location. This is clearly demonstrated by the data from coffin plates at St. Mary and St. Michael's which indicated that each grave cut for a stack of burials represented a single days work, rather than a family plot as might be assumed from the inclusion of adults of both sexes and children of all ages (Miles and Powers, 2006).

An overview of post-medieval burials in the capital demonstrates that differences in burial practice are predominantly socio-economic. For example, multiple internments in simple wooden boxes placed in long trench graves housed the poor of Somerstown (Powers and White in prep.), whilst generally, only the wealthier members of society could afford lead lined coffins or pay the premium for interment within brick vaults (Brickley and Buteaux, 2006: 154; Cox, 1996: 101; Curl, 2000: 40).

Poor Catholics ensured that their relatives were afforded a full funeral (Mayhew, 1851: 115), although burial within a Catholic cemetery was sometimes beyond their means (Garwood, 1853: 309). Examination of the documentary record may establish differences in the burial ceremony, laying out period and the tradition of holding a 'wake', but none of these factors are visible in the archaeological record alone.

In the predominantly Christian framework of the post-medieval period, it appears that there are no definitive identifiers for migrant groups within cemeteries, though socio-economic differences are observed and may elucidate other strands of evidence that suggest the presence of new population groups in an area.

Intrinsically linked to funerary practices is an examination of the material cultural of burial. Whether certain classes or styles of artefacts are cultural identifiers has been asked of the funerary evidence of many periods. Nixon *et al.* (2002: 72) identified the need for greater examination of the material culture of religious minorities and non-conformists in London, with a view to creating models which could then be used as interpretative tools. However, studies of artefacts from domestic contexts have recognised serious difficulties identifying cultural groups within post-medieval London (Jeffries, 2005). Within the graves at St. Mary and St. Michael, numerous crucifixes, including two particularly large crosses, four pendants of religious figures and several sets of rosary beads have also been identified. Perhaps the most surprising grave find was the recovery of an elaborate crucifix fashioned from a glazed white ceramic. This large piece consisted of a crucifix with a semicircular cup decorated with a lion's head below. It appears to have been designed to contain holy water and had fixings to allow it to be hung on a wall or other upright surface (Powell, 2006).

Such items might, therefore, be considered as cultural identifiers, indications of a religious difference signifying a culturally distinct group, yet few were found amongst the Catholic burials of St. Pancras. Here, just two examples were seen, a copper-alloy crucifix and pewter figure of Christ crucified (G. Egan, *pers. comm.*). It is suggested that this may indicate a temporal shift or changing fashions in certain grave inclusions.

This theory is supported by an apparently concurrent change in the predominant funeral attire. In the late 18th century, whilst some were buried in day clothes (Brickley *et al.,* 1999: 27), many of the dead were interred wearing shrouds or specifically made funerary dress, as seen in the burials at Christchurch, Spitalfields (Janaway, 1993: 95). Whilst some shroud pins were noted, leather shoes or boots, gloves and vast quantities of buttons from shirts, jackets and trousers indicate that most of the dead of this Whitechapel burial ground were interred fully clothed.

The adornment and symbolism of the burial container itself might enable the separation of cultural groups. Differences in religious imagery were noted in the external decoration of the coffins at St. Mary and St. Michael's compared with other, contemporary sites (A. Miles, *pers. comm.*). It appears that, in a period of widespread trade, coffin furniture and fittings may provide the most reliable artefactual clues to cultural or religious identity.

The osteological evidence: skeletal markers of 'difference'

Urbanisation, and particularly industrialisation, have been shown to have had a detrimental affect on human health, demonstrable by osteological analysis (Lewis, 2002). Migration is expected to increase levels of stress in those moving from rural to urban settlements, increasing susceptibility to disease and injury (Redfern and Roberts, 2005). The overcrowded, unsanitary living conditions of the poor in Victorian London certainly encouraged infectious disease, yet non-specific periostitis affected just 10% of the skeletal sample from St. Mary and St. Michael's, compared to more than 30% of the individuals at the Cross Bones burial ground Southwark (Brickley *et al.,* 1999), 16.9% (51/301) of the high status burials from St. Marylebone, Westminster (Miles *et al.,* in prep), and 15.8% (38/241) of those buried in the crypt of St. Luke's Old Street. A rate of 26.3% is cited for the period as a whole (Roberts and Cox, 2003: 344). It is possible that the data for St. Mary and St. Michael's are skewed by the high proportion of sub adults present. When the data for the adult population is examined alone, the prevalence rate of 18.4% (54/ 293), compares more closely to that of St. Marylebone at 19.7% (44/223), (Miles *et al.,* in prep) though it remains lower. Perhaps the apparently low prevalence represents an example of the 'osteological paradox' at work (Wood *et al.,* 1992)?

The observed rate of tuberculosis at St. Mary and St. Michael's (3/747: 0.4% or 3/293 adults: 1%), endemic in London during this time, was also lower than many contemporary sites (1.3% of individuals (4/301) and 1.3% of adults (3/223) were affected at St. Marylebone (Miles *et al.,* in prep)) but of a similar magnitude to the crude prevalence reported for the period: 0.5% (Roberts and Cox, 2003: 339).

Venereal syphilis, affecting 0.7% of the buried population (5/747) and 1.7% of the adults (5/293), was less frequent than the population prevalence at St. Brides Churchyard (1.1%) or the St. Pancras burial ground 1.7% (12/715), at the latter 2.3% (12/532) of adults were affected (Roberts and Cox, 2003: 341; Powers and White, in prep). Contemporary references refer to the chastity of the Irish Catholics in contrast to the native Londoners; young girls were chaperoned by their parents and adultery was uncommon (Garwood, 1853: 260; Mayhew, 1851: 109). Perhaps a behavioural difference influenced rates of infection, although the population prevalence of 0.7% is identical to that at St. Marylebone (2/301) where 0.9% (2/223) of adults were affected, and is not dissimilar to that seen for the period as a whole at 0.8% (Miles *et al.,* in prep; Roberts and Cox, 2003: 341).

Low rates of sub-adult enamel hypoplasia did not appear to reflect infant stress, but greater analysis of the relationship to age at death is required before firm conclusions can be drawn (Table 2). Cribra orbitalia was noted in 91 individuals from St. Mary and St. Michael's. The crude prevalence of 12.2% (91/747) compares closely with that seen at Christchurch Spitalfields (Roberts and Cox 2003: 307) and despite the high numbers of children at St. Mary and St. Michael's (such lesions remodel during later life) the prevalence is significantly lower than the 23.9% (72/301) seen in the high status St. Marylebone assemblage (Miles *et al.* in prep). The evidence of stress in the form of anaemia is, therefore, inconclusive.

Adult stature has been suggested as an indicator of environmental conditions and infant health, though the height attained as an adult is the result of both genetic and nutritional factors (Humphrey, 2000: 35). If the correlation between stature and relative nutritional status was strong, adult height differences could perhaps help identify migrant groups. Unfortunately, results from numerous post-medieval cemetery samples indicate no statistical difference in mean adult stature despite status differences (Miles *et al.,* in prep; Roberts and Cox, 2003; Boyle *et al.,* 2005).

The displaced agricultural labourers from Ireland often found work as hod carriers, excavators or dockers once in London, all of which involved heavy manual labour and increased risk of injury (Garwood, 1853: 315; Mayhew, 1851: 105). It appears that the London Irish also had a reputation for brawling (*ibid.*), although this may simply have been anti-Irish propaganda.

Table 2. Crude prevalence of enamel hypoplasia.

	Adult		Male		Female		Sub-adult		Total	
Observable dentitions	259		143		104		376		635	
	N	%	N	%	N	%	N	%	N	%
Enamel hypoplasia	29	11.2	19	13.3	10	9.6	4	1.1	33	5.2

At St. Mary and St. Michael's, 43 adults (14.7%) had evidence of healed long bone fractures. This rate lies within the range seen at other contemporary sites, though it is believed that further analysis may identify patterns in the type and location of injuries and the forces required to cause such trauma. For example, there were several instances of comminuted ankle fractures (Fig. 3). Twelve adult males (1.6% of the total assemblage: 12/747, 4% of adults: 12/293) displayed probable evidence of interpersonal violence. When compared to a crude overall prevalence of 4.7% (14/301, 6.3% of adults: 14/223) at St. Marylebone (Miles *et al.* in prep.) the rate actually suggests a group subject to *decreased* risk of assault.

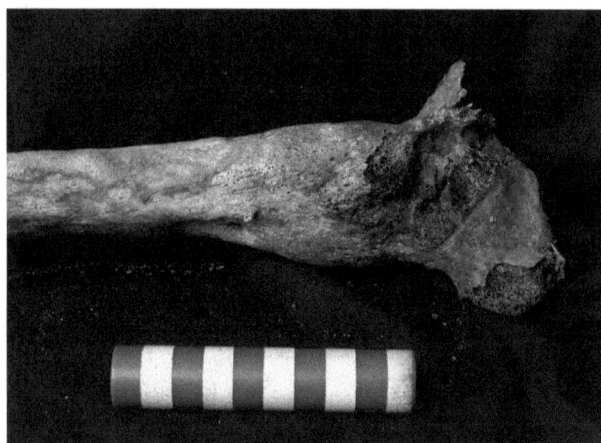

Figure 3. Comminuted ankle fracture with ankylosis: adult [1264] ©MoLAS.

Interestingly, examination of the burials from St. Mary and St. Michael showed that 22 males had notches in the anterior or lateral teeth resulting from the habitual use of a clay pipe (22/149: 14.8%) (Fig.4). No previous excavation has reported such a large number of cases: only one male from St. Marylebone (Miles *et al.*, in prep.) three men and a woman from the Cross Bones burial ground (Brickley *et al.*, 1999:34) and 11 individuals from St. Martin's (3.6%) (Brickley and Buteux, 2006:145) were affected. Whether this difference is temporal, cultural or status related is as yet unclear. Contemporary accounts certainly refer to the inhabitants of the East End as heavy smokers (Mayhew, 1851: 109).

Whilst it is evidently possible to identify differences both within and between cemetery populations using osteological data, the interpretation of the results is highly problematic. Even when examining a cemetery sample about which much is known, analysis requires the elimination of numerous social, and temporal, variables to establish the over-riding factor involved in the creation of any such difference. Since many pathological conditions are multi-factorial, establishing a definitive answer, or a pattern which signifies a largely migrant group, may be impossible.

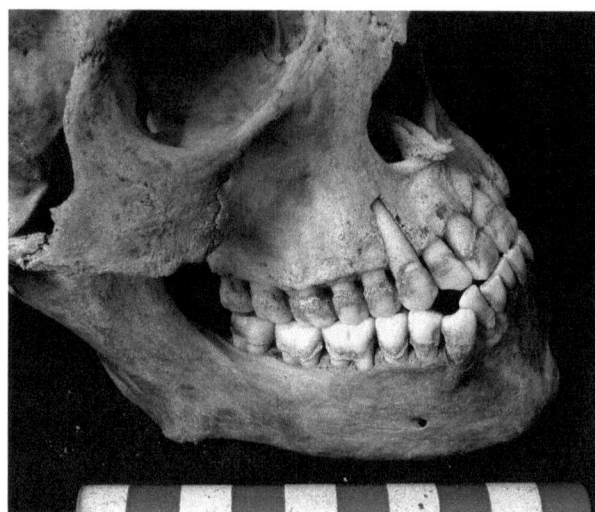

Figure 4. Pipe notch in the teeth of adult male [1268] – the left anterior teeth were also affected ©MoLAS.

The potential for isotopic analyses

Stable isotope analysis can demonstrate geographic mobility over the life course, and may provide information about childhood origins (Budd *et al.*, 2004: 127). This cemetery group may well contain 'first generation' adults and 'second generation' children: 72.2% of the sub-adults and 43.9% of the total population were less than 7 years old at the time of their death.

Oxygen isotopes have been used to indicate 'first generation' settlers and to establish their geographic origin (Budd *et al.*, 2004; Fricke *et al.*, 1995). The oxygen isotope ratio of rainwater (the ultimate source of drinking water) is related to climate as it varies with altitude, latitude and distance from the sea. Oxygen contained within skeletal tissues derives primarily from this drinking water (Bryant and Froelich, 1995: 4523). It therefore provides a record of the climatic zone in which people lived. In the British Isles, the oxygen isotope values of groundwater vary systematically from west to east (Darling *et al.*, 2003: 189). This presents the possibility of discriminating indigenous Londoners from immigrant settlers from many regions of Ireland (J. Montgomery, *pers. comm.*). Many of the Irish immigrants initially lived for some time in Bristol or Liverpool (Garwood, 1853: 256), but this would only be evident if the tooth chosen for analysis was mineralizing during this period of residence.

Strontium isotope ratios of body tissues relate to the uptake in the diet. Soil, plant and animal strontium ratios are linked to the underlying geology. This makes it possible to discriminate between people from different geographic areas, if these areas are geologically, and therefore isotopically, distinct (Price *et al.*, 2002, Bentley 2006). Much work still needs to be done to characterize different regions of Britain, but most of Ireland is geologically very different from the London region (J. Montgomery, *pers. comm.*). Strontium in bone and dentine is highly susceptible to diagenesis, but enamel appears to preserve lifetime values after burial (Trickett *et al.*, 2003: 653). In a post-medieval assemblage, it is possible that high rates of ante-mortem tooth loss could compromise scientific methods requiring dental enamel: at St. Mary and St. Michael, 70.7% of adults had lost one or more tooth during life. However, skeletal preservation of post-medieval assemblages is generally good, and the required sample size is small.

The use of oxygen and strontium isotopes in combination has been advocated as the most effective analytical tool, but since it is "technically difficult, labour intensive and expensive" (Budd *et al.*, 2004: 139) such work is likely to lie beyond the realms of most developer funded projects.

Since skeletal strontium is acquired through the diet, it is important to consider the origins of food during this period when meat was often raised some distance away from the Metropolis. This may also create difficulties if using animal proxies to examine background strontium values. However, although exotic imports entered London via the docks, documents suggest that the East End diet comprised mostly root vegetables and cheap meat (Garwood, 1853; Mayhew, 1851). Moreover, studies tend to conclude that skeletal strontium reflects the plant component of the diet, rather than meat and milk (Elias, 1980: 3).

The potential dietary differences between immigrants and the general population may also allow the study of carbon and nitrogen isotopes. A highly restricted diet, such as that suggested to have been widespread in the Irish lower classes at the time of the famine (Mayhew, 1851: 106), would produce a tight isotopic signal, and might allow differentiation from the background population. Comparison of values from dental and skeletal tissues could indicate dietary change over the life course and perhaps suggest geographic movement (J. Montgomery, *pers. comm.*).

In Britain, low-level contamination of the soil is seen in many areas, reflecting the long period of industrialisation. Lead may enter the diet through plants grown in and animals grazed on such soils. Modern studies have shown that lead concentrations are far greater in urban soils than in rural, agricultural areas (Thornton, 1998: 73-74). Many of the Irish migrants came to the Metropolis from the countryside. The quantity of lead in the teeth could be examined as it would be expected that those from rural Ireland would have lower values than a child born and raised in London (J. Montgomery, *pers. comm.*). Lead

absorbed by the human body comes from a variety of natural and anthropogenic sources. Lead piping and lead-tin solder used in plumbing for drinking water is one of the main sources of lead intake (Thornton, 1998: 73). Plumbing was in use in Victorian London, whilst the cottages of rural Ireland are more likely to have drawn their water directly from wells and so forth. Examination of the human remains from the ill-fated Franklin Expedition successfully demonstrated that the 19th century Europeans had lead levels much higher than the contemporary Inuit bone and equivalent to modern individuals exposed to high lead environments (Keenleyside *et al.*, 1997: 41).

The destructive analysis of human remains raises numerous ethical considerations. These are all the more acute for samples of relatively recent date, particularly where named individuals are recovered. It is vital that the scientific potential of the data justifies destructive work. Isotopic analysis requires only a small bone sample and a fragment of dental enamel. Innovation in the techniques used is constantly reducing the sample sizes required.

At the present time, most post-medieval skeletal assemblages are reburied shortly after osteological study. The scientific potential of hair should be considered, as retention of samples is unlikely to raise the same ethical objections as destructive testing of hard tissues. Although hair is recovered less frequently than skeletal material, in post-medieval burial assemblages a proportion of individuals with significant hair survival is not uncommon. At St. Mary and St. Michael, 27 burials contained hair (3.6%). Of these, 18 (2.4%) had only small quantities preserved, generally adjacent to copper alloy artefacts. In three cases the hair was sufficiently well preserved to enable observation of colour. Hair analysis can also provide high resolution information about the period immediately prior to the death of the individual (O'Connell and Hedges, 1999: 424).

Conclusions

Examination of the human remains from St. Mary and St. Michael demonstrates the problems that exist with the interpretation of cemetery assemblages. On a site where the geographic or cultural origins of many individuals are known or suspected, epigraphic evidence proved the only definitive indicator of migration. Although one could identify osteological patterns that differed from other, contemporary, sites it was not possible to recognise immigrant groups or individuals. This is highly problematic since the quantity of epigraphic data is often limited, even in large post-medieval excavations.

It is only with large-scale scientific analyses that the issue of migration and osteological indicators of difference can be effectively addressed. Given the wealth of circumstantial evidence and documentary evidence of life in Victorian Whitechapel, the cemetery population from St. Mary and St. Michael would make an ideal test case: utilising a group of individuals where many of the, usually unknown, variables can be quantified. Theoretical questions common to all cemetery assemblages could be studied using data acquired from post-medieval groups. As Nixon *et al.* (2002: 71) stated, models established using historic cemetery populations have great potential as interpretative tools for earlier, non-documented populations.

Acknowledgements

The author wishes to thank the Archdiocese of Westminster for funding work at St. Mary and St. Michael, Tracy Wellman, Andy Chopping and Maggie Cox for providing illustrations, Adrian Miles, particularly for his help with historical references, Robin Wroe-Brown and the excavation team, Dr Janet Montgomery for her correspondence on the use of stable isotopes, Martin Smith for his patience, and the editors and reviewers whose comments were of great help in improving the original draft of this paper.

Bibliography

Bentley, R.A. 2006. "Strontium isotopes from the earth to the archaeological skeleton: a review". *Journal of Archaeological Method and Theory* 13: 135-187.

Boyle, A., Boston, C. and Witkin, A. 2005. *The Archaeological Experience at St. Luke's Church, Old Street, Islington.* Oxford Archaeology, (unpublished).

Brickley, M. and Miles, A. with Stainer, H. 1999. *The Cross Bones Burial Ground Redcross Way Southwark London: Archaeological Excavations (1991-1998) for the London Underground Limited Jubilee Line Extension Project.* London: MoLAS Monograph 3.

Brickley, M. and Buteux, S. and Adams, J. and Cherrington, R. 2006. *St. Martin's Uncovered: Investigations in the Churchyard of St. Martin's-in-the-Bull Ring, Birmingham, 2001* Oxford: Oxbow.

Bryant, J.D. and Froelich, P.N. 1995. "A model of oxygen isotope fractionation in body water of large mammals". *Geochimica et Cosmochimica Acta* 59: 4523-4537.

Budd, P., Millard, A., Chenery, A., Lucy, S. and Roberts, C. 2004. "Investigating population movement by stable isotope analysis: a report from Britain" *Antiquity* 78: 127-141.

Census Finder –Irish Clans and Surnames (www.censusfinder.com/irish-surnames.htm) accessed July 2006.

Cox, M. 1996. *Life and death in Spitalfields 1700-1850.* York: Council for British Archaeology.

Cox, M. and Mays, S. (eds.) 2000. *Human Osteology in Archaeology and Forensic Science.* London: Greenwich Medical Media.

Curl, J.S. 2000. *The Victorian celebration of death.* Stroud: Sutton Publishing.

Darling, W.G., Bath, A.H. and Talbot, J.C. 2003. "The O and H stable isotopic composition of fresh waters in the British Isles: 2, Surface waters and groundwater" *Hydrology and Earth System Sciences* 7:183-195.

Elias, M. 1980. "The feasibility of dental strontium analysis for diet-assessment of human populations" *American Journal of Physical Anthropology* 53: 1-4.

Garwood, J. 1853. *The Million Peopled City.* London: Wertheim and Macintosh.

Grauer, A.L., McNamara, E.M. and Houdek, D.V. 1998. "A history of their own: patterns of death in a nineteenth-century poorhouse". In: Grauer, A.L. and Stuart-Macadam, P. (eds.) *Sex and Gender in Palaeopathological Perspective.* Cambridge: Cambridge University Press. 149-164.

Humphrey, L. 2000. "Growth studies of past populations: an overview and an example". In Cox, M. and Mays, S. (eds.) *Human Osteology in Archaeology and Forensic Science.* London: Greenwich Medical Media. 23-38.

Jackson, L. 2006. *A Dictionary of Victorian London.* London: Anthem Press.

Janaway, R.C. 1993. "The textiles". In: Reeves, J and Adams, M. *The Spitalfields Project. Volume 1: The Archaeology - Across the Styx.* CBA Research Report No 85. 93-119.

Jeffries, N. 2005. "Material histories of 19th-century Londoners: telling new tales of the Metropolis" *Friends News*, Museum of London, July–September, 10–11.

Keenleyside, A., Bertulli, M. and Fricke, H.C. 1997. "The final days of the Franklin Expedition: new skeletal evidence" *Arctic* 50: 36-46.

Lewis, M.E. 2002. "The impact of industrialisation: comparative study of child health in four sites from medieval and post-medieval England (850-1859)" *American Journal of Physical Anthropology* 119: 211-223.

Mayhew, H. 1851. *London Labour and the London Poor: The condition and earnings of those that will work, those that cannot work and those that will not work, Vol. 1.* London: Charles Griffen and Co.

McDonnell, K.G.T. 1969. "Roman Catholics in London". In: Hollaender, A.E.J. and Kellaway, W. (eds) *Studies in London History.* London: Hodder and Stoughton. 429–45.

Miles, A. and Powers, N. 2006. *Bishop Challoner Catholic Collegiate School, Lukin Street, London, E1: a post-excavation assessment and updated project design.* MoLAS (unpublished).

Miles, A., Powers, N., Wroe-Brown, R. with Walker, D. (in prep.) *St. Marylebone Church and Burial Ground: Excavations at St. Marylebone Church of England School, 2005.* London: MoLAS.

Montgomery, J. 2002. "Lead and Strontium Isotope Compositions of Human Dental Tissues as an Indicator of Ancient Exposure and Population Dynamics". PhD thesis, University of Bradford.

Murphy, M. 1991. *Catholic poor schools in Tower Hamlets (London) 1765–1865: Part 1 Wapping and Commercial Road.* London: M. Murphy.

Nixon, T. *et al.* 2002. *A Research Framework for London Archaeology.* London: Museum of London.

O'Connell, T.C. and Hedges, R.E.M. 1999. "Investigations into the effect of diet on modern human hair isotopic values" *American Journal of Physical Anthropology* 108: 409-425.

Pollard, T.M. and Hyatt, S.B. 1999. "Sex, gender and health: integrating biological and social perspectives". In: Pollard, T.M. and Hyatt, S.B. (eds.) *Sex, Gender and Health.* Cambridge: Cambridge University Press Biosocial Society Symposium Series. 1-17.

Powell, N. 2006. "The accessioned finds". In: Miles, A. and Powers, N. *Bishop Challoner Catholic Collegiate School, Lukin Street, London, E1: a post-excavation assessment and updated project design.* MoLAS (unpublished).

Powers, N. and White, W. (in prep.) "Health and Disease". In: Emery, P.A. and Wooldridge, K. *Channel Tunnel Rail Link New London Terminus: Archaeological investigations in St. Pancras burial ground 2002-3.* London: MoLAS.

Price, T.D., Burton, J.H. and Bentley, R.A. 2002. "The characterization of biologically available strontium isotope ratios for the study of prehistoric migration". *Archaeometry.* 44: 117-135.

Redfern, R.C. and Roberts, C.A. 2005. "Health in Romano-British Urban Communities: Reflections from the Cemeteries". In: Smith, D., Brickley, M. and Smith, W. (eds.) *Fertile Ground: Papers in Honour of Susan Limbrey.* Association for Environmental Archaeology Symposia No. 22. Oxford: Oxbow Books. 115-129.

Roberts, C.A. and Cox, M. 2003. *Health and Disease in Britain: from prehistory to the present day.* Stroud: Sutton Publishing.

Rousham, E.K. 1999. "Gender bias in South Asia: effects on child growth and nutritional status". In: Pollard, T.M. and Brin Hyatt, S. (eds.) *Sex, Gender and Health.*

Biosocial Society Symposium Series. Cambridge: Cambridge University Press. 37-52.

Rousham, E.K. and Humphrey, L.T. 2002. "The dynamics of child survival". In: Macbeth, H. and Collinson, P. (eds.). *Human population dynamics: cross-disciplinary perspectives.* Biosocial Society Symposium Series. Cambridge: Cambridge University Press. 124-140.

Sherwell, A. 1897. *Life in West London: A Study and a Contrast.* London: Methuen.

Thornton, I. 1998. "Trends in environmental lead levels: implications for human exposure". In: Gompertz, D. (ed.) *IEH report on recent UK blood lead surveys.* Medical Research Council, Institute for Environment and Health Report R9. Leicester: Institute for Environment and Health. 67-84.

Trickett, M.A., Budd, P., Montgomery, J. and Evans, J. 2003. "An assessment of solubility profiling as a decontamination procedure for the Sr-87/Sr-86 analysis of archaeological human skeletal tissue" *Applied Geochemistry* 18: 653-658.

Walker, P.L. 1995. "Biases in preservation and sexism in sexing: some lessons from historical collections for the paleodemographers". In: Saunders, S.R. and Herring, A. (eds.) *Grave Reflections: portraying the past through cemetery studies.* Toronto: Canadian's Scholar's Press Inc. 31-47.

Westminster Diocesan Archive, R/74, letter dated 5th December 1853.

Wood, J.W., Milner, G.R., Harpending, H. and Weiss, K.M. 1992. "The Osteological Paradox: problems of inferring prehistoric health from skeletal samples" *Current Anthropology* 33: 343-370.

Periapical voids in human jaw bones

Alan R. Ogden

Biological Anthropology Research Centre, Archaeological Sciences, University of Bradford, Bradford, West Yorkshire, BD7 1DP

e-mail address for correspondence: arogden@bradford.ac.uk

Abstract

This paper attempts to clarify the different types of apical voids that may be found in human jaws. It distinguishes between granulomata, granulomata with cyst development and chronic abscesses, but concludes that although these stressed the individual's immune system, they probably caused relatively little pain or discomfort in the long-term. In archaeological populations, eruption of teeth, to compensate for the high tooth wear, led to most root apices becoming more superficial by middle life, and this too helped to lessen the impact of their apical pathology. The size of the void, its surface lining and its interface with the cortical bone of the maxilla or mandible give valuable clues as to the nature of the original lesion. Radiographs are essential to identify otherwise hidden voids, especially in mandibles.

Keywords: dental; periapical; granuloma; cyst; abscess

Introduction

Periapical voids seen in jaws from archaeological collections are often dramatic (Figs. 1a, b.). They are variously described in the literature as abscesses, cysts, granulomata, fenestrations, dehiscences, or other more esoteric terms (Bhaskar, 1966; Lineberg et al., 1972; Linn et al., 1987; Nair, 2004; Chazel and Mafart, 2004). Dias and Tayles (1997), in a seminal paper that did not attract the attention it deserved, highlighted the need for much greater precision of diagnosis and this paper is an attempt to supply that.

Fenestration simply means an opening, from the Latin *fenestra*, a window. It says nothing about the possible cause or pathology involved. Dehiscence is often used to describe tooth roots exposed to view, not because of pathology, but because the overlying paper-thin bone has been lost by taphonomic processes. A word relating to seeds, strictly speaking it means a "gaping or a bursting open", and so is not appropriate. Dento-alveolar lesions in the jaws have until recently been described routinely in osteological reports as "abscesses" with all that this implies about pain, infection and general health (Dias and Tayles, 1997; Hillson, 2005: 307-314). Extensive modern clinical and histological studies indicate however that such voids are relatively common, are usually painless granulomata, and fewer than a third of them may be actually infected (Table 1).

The vast majority of regions of apical bone loss, found in modern-day patients by radiographs, are completely painless and 40% of pulps which become necrotic may do so without any symptoms (Michaelson and Holland, 2002). Most develop completely symptom-free apical granulomata following pulp death and aseptic autolysis. A few larger granulomata, with rounded and clearly defined sclerotic margins may have undergone cystic change, slowly expanding, again without symptoms. Some are periapical abscesses long past their acute and painful stage, having developed chronic drainage through sinuses or along the periodontal ligament. Quiescent granulomata, cysts or chronic abscesses can, however, be stirred into acute activity by new pulpal or blood-borne infection, or by a reduction in host immune response due to illness, stress or malnutrition.

Table 1. Histological analysis of soft-tissue lesions related to root apices. Several of these researchers did not consider they could clearly distinguish between granulomata and abscesses and so did not record abscesses separately.

Authors	n.	Granulomata	Cysts	Abscesses
Nakade et al. 1989	91	54%	46%	na
Spatafore et al. 1990	1659	52%	42%	na
Nobuhara & del Rio 1993	150	59%	22%	na
Ramachadran Nair et al. 1996	256	50%	15%	35%
Sanchis et al. 1998	125	86%	14%	na
Kuc et al. 2000	788	51%	47%	2%
Vier & Figuerdo 2002	104	na	24%	64%
Ricucci et al. 2006 a	50	40%	32%	28%
Ricucci et al. 2006 b	60	78%	15%	na

Granulomata and cysts

To understand the formation of a granuloma it is essential to realise that the dental pulp in a mature tooth has virtually no ability to repair itself when damaged, whether by trauma, caries or exposure to the oral environment. Its blood supply arrives through very narrow channels in the root, and any inflammation in the virtually sealed pulp chamber increases the internal pressure, occludes the blood supply and leads to the death of the pulp. The necrotic pulp then undergoes autolysis, which will be sterile if bacteria or fungi cannot gain access. The concomitant release of breakdown products from the necrotic pulp elicits an inflammatory response (either acute or chronic) from the soft tissues surrounding the apex of the tooth. This soft tissue lesion, a periapical granuloma, is a sphere of soft tissue surrounding the root apex and it creates a space in the surrounding bone (Cawson *et al.*, 2002: 60-61). It is this space that is seen in osteological specimens or radiographs and that we need to interpret. If there is a bony cavity related to a tooth apex, it reveals for certain that the dental pulp, or at

the very least, the pulp in that particular root, must have been dead for some time, even if there is no obvious sign of trauma or disease in the tooth itself.

The essential components of a granuloma are collections of modified macrophages, usually with a surrounding zone of lymphocytes. Granulomatous inflammation seems to require the presence of indigestible or constantly replenished foreign material. In the case of dental granulomata, it would seem that breakdown products continue to leak from the apex, as polymorphs are unable to access the necrotic pulp chamber and remove its contents. Granulomata from different roots may eventually become confluent, forming larger areas. The central areas of inflammation often undergo necrosis as they become remote from their blood supply. This leads to the formation of cystic spaces within them which undergo slow enlargement over a period of years, as osmotic pressure leads to fluid build-up in the interior and as they become lined by membrane developed from the epithelial cell rests of Malassez (Cawson *et al.*, 2002: 104; Nanci, 2003: 106; Ricucci *et al.*, 2006b). The increasing hydrostatic pressure leads periodontal cysts to expand at approximately 5mm in diameter per year (Soames and Southam, 1998), unless the tooth is completely removed, and they may eventually become very large (Fig. 1b). Thus some extensive lesions are hybrid in nature, so that, for example, one region of the lesion may still be a simple granuloma while another may show signs of cyst or chronic abscess formation (Ricucci *et al.*, 2006a).

Abscesses

A necrotic pulp and granuloma/cyst is highly likely to become infected, either through contamination from the mouth or by blood-borne infection (Trowbridge and Stevens, 1992; Abbott, 2002, 2004). In the absence of a smooth-walled sinus tracking out through the cortical bone, which indicates the presence of a chronic abscess, all that can be proved by the presence of an apical void is that the tooth was non-vital. Whether or not it was causing pain at the time of death is impossible to tell. An acute abscess rapidly invades trabecular spaces and vascular channels, but may not form a bone cavity because there is insufficient time for osteoclastic resorption. The pus tracks through bone, taking the path of least resistance, until it reaches an outer surface where it discharges (Dias and Tayles, 1997). These convoluted, multiple and narrow pathways are difficult to identify *in vivo*, let alone in dry bone, as they do not show on radiographs. However, the presence of a visible buccal or lingual sinus in the bone is evidence that, at some time, there was a painful abscess which has since drained and become chronic (Hillson, 2005: 307-314). A typical chronic abscess is shown in Figure 2.

Upper posterior teeth sometimes drain into the maxillary antrum and may lead to the formation of a chronic oro-antral fistula. Lower molars can also, rarely, drain through the vertical ramus of the mandible leading to a particularly painful and intractable sub-masseteric

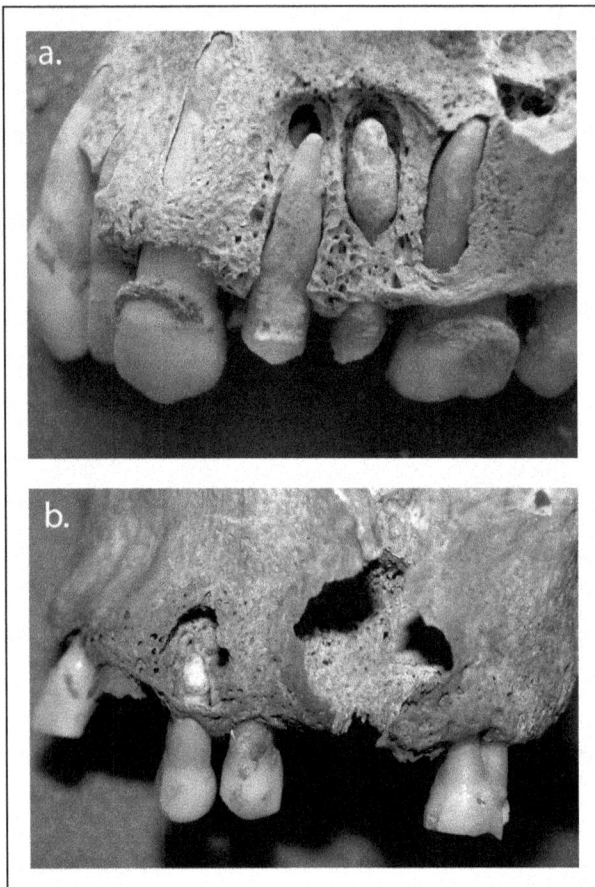

Figure 1. a.) Left maxilla of an individual from Medieval Hereford, with a variety of holes in the alveolus. Large globular spaces above the premolar roots show that these teeth were non-vital and in life had dental granulomata wrapped around their apices. There are no such spaces above the apices of the canine, incisors or molar, showing that the pulps of these teeth were vital. Their roots have only been exposed by taphonomic damage of the cortical plate of the alveolus, and there is no apical pathology. b.) Left maxilla of an individual from the battle of Towton 1461. The upper left first premolar has a moderately large apical granuloma, probably becoming cystic because of its size. The lost upper left first molar had a large periapical cyst (note the lack of porosity, indicating the presence of a lining membrane). The grossly carious upper left canine has not however developed a visible apical granuloma, either because the thickness of the overlying bone masks it, or because the infection could drain freely down the pulp canal.

abscess, as illustrated in Figure 3. Also, whenever a single tooth has developed greater periodontal destruction than any of its neighbours, or its contralateral equivalent, pulp death with pus drainage along the periodontal ligament should be suspected as the primary cause (Clarke and Hirsch, 1991; Dias and Tayles, 1997).

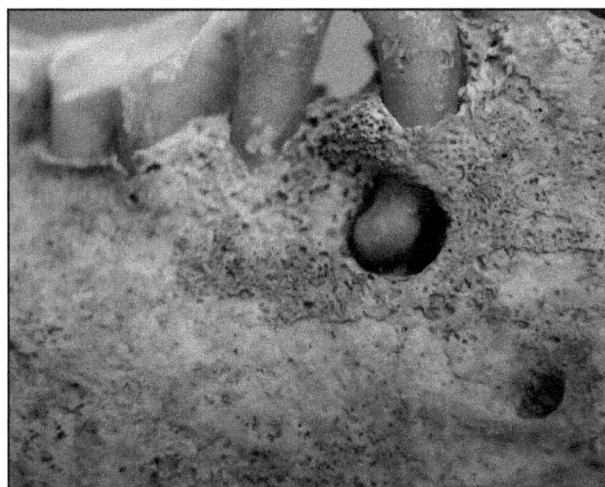

Figure 2. Typical chronic abscess, on the mesial root of a lower first molar whose pulp has been exposed by severe attrition. The edge of the bone cavity is rounded and thickened distally and there is formation of a plaque of new bone over the surrounding surface.

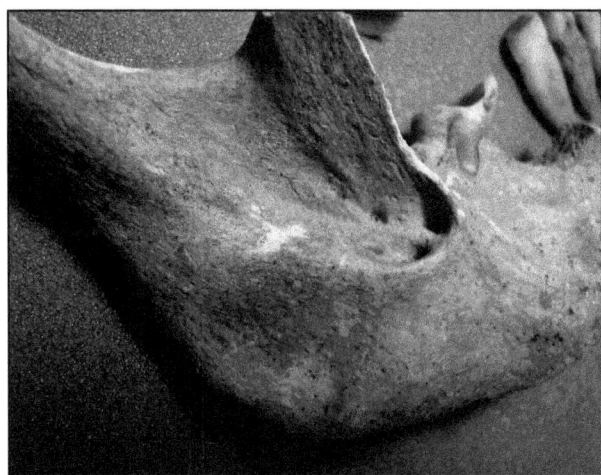

Figure 3. Submasseteric abscess, this is a view of the buccal aspect of the right mandible of individual 1259 from Mediaeval Hereford. A chronic infection from the lower third molar had for years been draining beneath the masseter muscle cf. Jones *et al.*, 2003. Note the smooth and rounded contour of the double sinus, indicating repeated bony remodelling.

Newman and Levers (1979) and Levers and Darling (1983) demonstrated eruption compensating for attrition in archaeological skulls and Clarke and Hirsch (1991) proved, using the inferior dental canal as a fixed point, that coronal movement of the tooth to compensate for wear was relative to the investing tissues and resulted in the teeth moving coronally past a vertically stable periodontium. With the severe wear common in most archaeological populations, teeth became relatively superficial in the jaws by middle life, and this too probably served to lessen the impact of their apical pathology.

Differential diagnosis

There have been reports in the literature over the years of attempts to make a differential diagnosis between cyst and granuloma based on their size and radiological features. Cysts are considered to be larger than granulomata, and if the lesion is greater than 15mm in diameter it would certainly be considered a cyst (Mortensen *et al.*, 1970; Whaites, 1992; Goaz *and* White, 1994; Ledesma-Montes *et al.*, 2000). However Dias and Tayles (1997) and Dias *et al.* (2007) consider that any void greater than 3mm in diameter is probably cystic. A cyst was thought in the past to exhibit defined margins with a thin radio-opaque border whereas a granuloma would show indistinct margins (Shear, 1976; Gallego-Romero *et al.*, 2002). However recent studies (Reit *et al.*, 2003; Ricucci *et al.*, 2006a) comparing radiological diagnosis with histological diagnosis, show that there appears to be no correlation between the two, presumably because the radiography is so affected by the structure of the overlying bone.

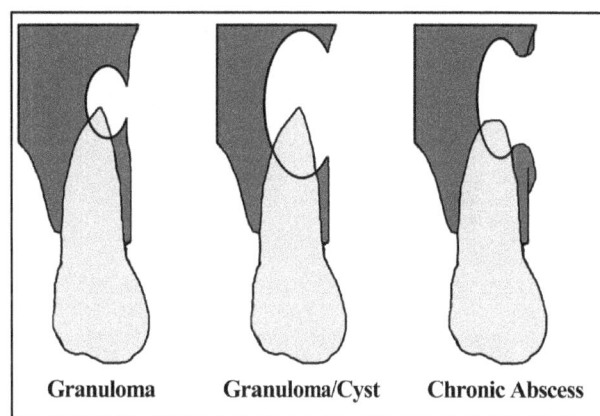

Figure 4. The basic characteristics of granuloma, granuloma/cyst, and chronic abscess. The granuloma and granuloma/cyst are exposed by taphonomic damage to the overlying eggshell thickness of bone, displaying a sharp edge. The chronic abscess has a rolled and thickened rim where it penetrates the cortical plate of the alveolus, and the opening is surrounded by a "halo" of new bone deposition. The lining of the void is porous for the passage of blood vessels in granulomata and abscesses, but less so in cysts, which develop a lining membrane.

Large scale histological studies of soft-tissue lesions on the apices of extracted teeth have indicated a wide range of diagnoses (Table 1). All workers agree that the most common lesions are best described histologically as granulomata, but the percentages present varied from 40% to 86%. Cyst development had occurred somewhere in the lesion in 15-47% of cases. There were however

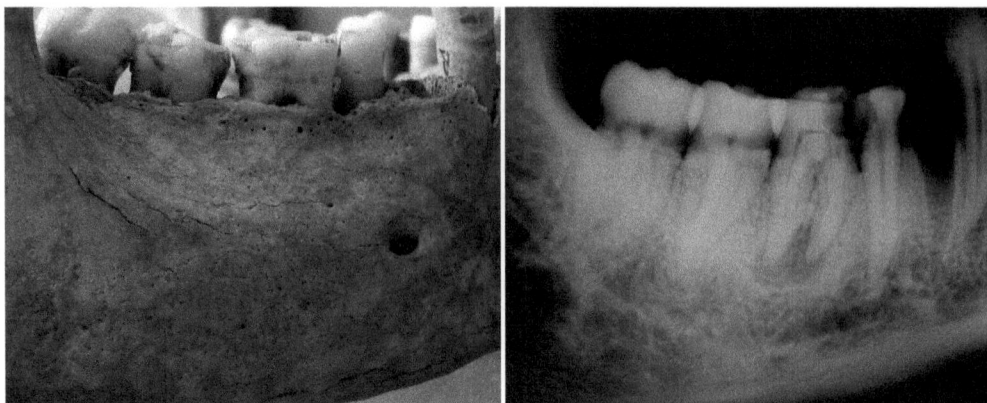

Figure 5. This mandible shows no apparent alveolar lesion, but a radiograph reveals a large periapical void at the roots of the first molar, distal to the mental foramen. This emphasises the importance of radiological examination of mandibles, the dense cortical bone of which can easily mask large lesions.

major disagreements about whether abscesses could be clearly identified. These pathologists have confirmed the difficulty of making a differential diagnosis even if the histology is available, let alone simply from the gross or radiographic morphology of the periapical void in the bone. For that reason palaeopathologists can only make tentative judgements as to the likely diagnosis of voids in alveoli.

When examining voids in dry maxillae or mandibles, there are several characteristics to look for in order to aid diagnosis (Fig. 4).

1. If the void is a granuloma it is usually 2-3mm in diameter and is smoothly rounded in shape. Voids larger than 3mm in diameter are more likely to be developing internal cysts (Dias and Tayles, 1997; Dias *et al.*, 2007).

2. The lesion must extend from, or incorporate the apices of, one or more tooth roots. If it does not clearly involve the apex of the tooth it may involve an accessory or lateral root canal, (Clarke and Hirsch, 1991). If not closely related to a root it is more likely to be a local manifestation of a systemic disease e.g. multiple myeloma or metastatic carcinoma, and there will probably be similar lesions elsewhere in the skeleton.

3. The lining of a void is smooth but porous, allowing access for the copious blood supply. The less the porosity of the void wall, the greater the chance of it having developed into a cyst and having developed a lining membrane.

4. A void with a thin, sharp margin where it meets the cortical surface of the alveolus indicates the presence of a non-infected granuloma or cyst. If the margin is rounded or thickened and the bone appears to have been frequently remodelled, often with a halo of new bone around the orifice, then this represents a chronic abscess, which would have been seeping pus for a considerable time.

Previous osteological studies indicate that granulomata are more common in the maxilla than the mandible and explain this by the greater complexity of the upper root forms (Bhaskar, 1966; Lineberg, 1972; Linn *et al.*, 1987; Kieser *et al.*, 2001; Nair, 2004). However, it may be also because the thick cortical bone of the mandible conceals voids much more effectively than the more porous bone of the maxilla. Without radiographs many mandibular defects, and thus non-vital teeth, are missed (Fig. 5). Radiographs are therefore essential if the true picture of dental health in a community is to be assessed (Rushton *et al.*, 2002). However it must be remembered that the radiographic appearance will not authoritatively distinguish between granulomata and cysts (Ricucci *et al.*, 2006b).

Conclusions

If there is a bony cavity related to a tooth apex, it reveals for certain that the dental pulp, or at the very least, the pulp in that particular root, must have been dead for some time, even if there is no obvious sign of trauma or disease. This paper has built on the important work of Dias and Tayles (1997) and attempts to clarify the different types of apical voids that may be found in the jaws. It distinguishes between granulomata, granuloma/cysts and chronic abscesses. Extensive modern clinical and histological studies indicate however that such voids are relatively common, are usually painless granulomata, and fewer than a third of them may be actually infected. In archaeological populations, eruption of teeth, to compensate for the high tooth wear, led to most root apices becoming more superficial by middle life, and this helped to lessen the impact of their apical pathology. This paper concludes that although these lesions placed a burden upon the individual's immune system, they probably caused less pain or distress in the long-term, than has been assumed. If a true comparison between the incidences of maxillary and mandibular periapical voids is to be made, radiographs are essential to identify otherwise hidden voids, especially in mandibles.

Acknowledgements

The author would like to thank Jane Martin who helped to present the original poster at the BABAO Conference 2004 which led to the production of this paper.

Literature cited

Abbott, P.V. 2002. "The periapical space - a dynamic interface" *Australian Endodontic Journal* 28: 96-107.

Abbott, P.V. 2004. "Classification, diagnosis and clinical manifestations of apical periodontitis" *Endodontic Topics* 8: 36.

Bhaskar, S.N. 1966. "Periapical lesions – types, incidence and clinical features" *Oral Surgery, Oral Medicine, Oral Pathology, Oral Radiology and Endodontics* 21: 657-668.

Cawson, R.A., Odell, E. and Porter, S. 2002. *Essentials of oral pathology and oral medicine*. Edinburgh: Churchill Livingstone.

Chazel, J-C. and Mafart, B. 2004. "Apical lesions" *British Dental Journal* 196: 2-3.

Clarke, N.G. and Hirsch, R.S. 1991. "Physiological, pulpal and periodontal factors influencing alveolar bone". In: Kelly, M.A. and Larsen, C.S. (eds.) *Advances in Dental Anthropology*. New York, Willey-Liss. 241-266.

Dias G. and Tayles, N. 1997. "Abscess cavity: a misnomer" *International Journal of Osteoarchaeology* 7: 548-554.

Dias, G., Prasad, K. and Santos, A.L. 2007. "Pathogenesis of apical periodontal cysts: Guidelines for diagnosis in paleopathology" *International Journal of Osteoarchaeology* (in press- published online 11/04/2007 www.interscience.wiley.com DOI: 10.1002/oa.902).

Gallego Romero, D., Torres Lagares, D., Garcia Calderon, M., Romero Ruiz, M.M., Infante Cossio, P. and Gutierrez Perez, J.L. 2002. "Differential diagnosis and therapeutic approach to periapical cysts in daily dental practice" *Medicina Oral* 7: 59-62.

Goaz, P.W. and White, S.C. 1994. *Oral Radiology: Principles and interpretation*. St Louis: C.V. Mosby.

Hillson, S. 2005. *Teeth*. 2nd edition. Cambridge: Cambridge University Press.

Jones, K.C., Silver, J., Millar, W.S. and Mandel, L. 2003. "Chronic submasseteric abscess: anatomic, radiologic, and pathologic features" *American Journal of Neuroradiology* 24: 1159-1163.

Kieser, J.A., Kelsen, A., Love, R., Herbison, P.G.P. and Dennison, K.J. 2001. "Periapical lesions and dental wear in the early Maori" *International Journal of Osteoarchaeology* 11: 290-297.

Kuc, I., Peters, E. and Pan, J. 2000. "Comparison of clinical and histologic diagnoses in periapical lesions" *Oral Surgery, Oral Medicine, Oral Pathology, Oral Radiology and Endodontics* 89: 333-7.

Ledesma-Montes, C., Hernadez-Guerro, J.C. and Garces-Ortiz, M. 2000. "Clinico-pathologic study of odontogenic cysts in a Mexican sample population" *Archives of Medical Research* 31: 373-376.

Levers, R.G.H. and Darling, A.I. 1983. "Continuing eruption of some adult human teeth of ancient populations" *Archives of Oral Biology* 28: 401-8.

Lineberg, W.B., Waldron, C.A. and Delanne, G.F. 1972. "A clinical, roentgenographic and histopathologic evaluation of periapical lesions" *Oral Surgery, Oral Medicine, Oral Pathology* 17: 467.

Linn, J., Srikandi, W., Clarke, N. and Smith, T. 1987. "Radiographic and visual assessment of alveolar pathology in first molars in dry skulls" *American Journal of Physical Anthropology* 72: 515-521.

Michaelson, P.L. and Holland, G.R. 2002. "Is pulpitis painful?" *International Endodontic Journal.* 35: 829-832.

Mortensen, H., Winther, J.E. and Birn, H. 1970. "Periapical granulomas and cysts. An investigation of 1600 cases" *Scandinavian Journal of Dental Research* 78: 241-250.

Nair, P.N. 2004. "Pathogenesis of apical periodontitis and the causes of endodontic failures" *Critical Reviews in Oral Biology and Medicine* 15: 348-381.

Nakade, O., Ohuchi, T., Seki, C., Kanno, H., Abe, H., Kaku, T. and Okuyama, T. 1989. "Survey of histopathological services in the Department of Oral Pathology, Higashi-Nippon-Gakuen University, 1979-1989" *Higashi Nippon Shigaku Zasshi* 8: 39-46.

Nanci, A. 2003. *Ten Cate's Oral Histology: Development, Structure and Function.* St Louis: Mosby.

Newman, H.N. and Levers, B. 1979. "Tooth eruption and function in an early Anglo-Saxon population" *Journal of the Royal Society of Medicine* 72: 341-350.

Nobuhara, W.K. and del Rio, C.E. 1993. "Incidence of periradicular pathoses in endodontic treatment failures" *Journal of Endodontics* 19: 315-318.

Ramachadran Nair, P.N., Pajarola, G. and Schroeder, H.E. 1996. "Types and incidence of human periapical lesions obtained with extracted teeth" *Oral Surgery, Oral Medicine, Oral Pathology, Oral Radiology and Endodontics* 81: 93-102.

Reit, C., Petersson, K. and Molven, O. 2003. "Diagnosis of pulpal and periapical disease". In: Bergenholtz, G., Hørsted-Bindslev, P. and Reit, C. (eds.) *Textbook of Endodontology*. Oxford: Blackwell Munksgaard. 9-18.

Ricucci, D., Pascon, E.A., Pitt Ford, T.R. and Langeland, K. 2006a "Epithelium and bacteria in periapical lesions". *Oral Surgery, Oral Medicine, Oral Pathology, Oral Radiology and Endodontics* 101: 239-249.

Ricucci, D., Mannocci, F., and Ford, T.R. 2006b. "A study of periapical lesions correlating the presence of a radiopaque lamina with histological findings" *Oral Surgery, Oral Medicine, Oral Pathology, Oral Radiology and Endodontics* 101: 389-394.

Rushton, V.E., Horner, K. and Worthington, H.V. 2002. "Routine panoramic radiography of new adult patients in general dental practice: relevance of diagnostic yield to treatment and identification of radiographic selection criteria" *Oral Surgery, Oral Medicine, Oral Pathology, Oral Radiology and Endodontics* 93: 488-495.

Sanchis, J.M., Penarrocha, M., Bagan, M., Guarinos, J. and Vera, F. 1998. "Incidence of radicular cysts in a series of 125 chronic periapical lesions" *Revue de Stomatologie et de Chirurgie Maxillo-Faciale* 98: 354-358.

Shear, M. 1976. *Cysts of the oral regions*. Bristol: John Wright.

Soames, J.V. and Southam, J.C. 1998. *Oral pathology*. New York: Oxford University Press.

Spatafore, C.M., Griffin, J.A., Keyes, G.G., Wearden, S. and Skidmore, A.E. 1990. "Periapical biopsy report: an analysis of over a 10-year period" *Journal of Endodontics* 16: 239-241.

Trowbridge, H.O. and Stevens, B.H. 1992. "Microbiologic and pathologic aspects of pulpal and periapical disease" *Current Opinion in Dentistry* 2: 85-92.

Vier, F.V. and Figueirdo, J.A. 2002. "Prevalence of different periapical lesions associated with human teeth and their correlation with the presence and extension of apical external root resorption" *International Endodontic Journal* 35: 710-719.

Whaites, E. 1992. *Essentials of Dental Radiography and Radiology*. Edinburgh: Churchill Livingstone.

Great Chesterford: a catalogue of burials

Sarah Inskip

School of Humanities (Archaeology), Avenue Campus, University of Southampton,
Southampton, SO17 1BF
e-mail address for correspondence: sai204@soton.ac.uk

Abstract

A series of excavations of the Anglo-Saxon cemetery at Great Chesterford (Essex) were undertaken between 1952 and 1955. The excavation report indicates that 161 graves were identified within the cemetery containing 167 inhumations. Furthermore, 31 deposits of cremated bone and a series of animal burials were also recovered.

Although previous analysis has been conducted (Waldron, 1994), problems of curation mean that the collection's research potential has not been fully realised. At the University of Southampton a new process of reorganising and cataloguing the collection has been undertaken. As part of this, preliminary analysis of the collection has begun. This paper aims to highlight the research potential of the skeletal material by describing the work undertaken so far, which includes developing a complete inventory. A comparison with the original report and a brief description of unreported pathologies is also provided. Notable features include a high level of infant recovery and significant levels of infectious disease, potentially tuberculosis.

Keywords: Anglo-Saxon, cemetery, curation, Essex, juvenile

Introduction

The bones of 161 graves comprising 167 inhumations have been studied and re-analysed. The remains derive from the Anglo-Saxon cemetery dating to AD 450 – 600. The cemetery itself is located north west of the Roman town of Great Chesterford (OS grid no.TL 501435 – Fig.1). Some of the remains have been damaged by gravel digging and ploughing (Evison, 1994). Many burials contained a few stray animal bones and there are instances of unassociated disarticulated human bone. Thirty one deposits of cremated bone were also found, in addition to two horse and two dog burials (although these are not discussed in this paper).

The human remains from Great Chesterford were received from English Heritage by the University of Southampton in the summer of 2004. Although mostly labelled, the elements were boxed by element, rather than by discrete individual. The labelled skeletal material was reorganised back into individuals, but problems arose when trying to identify the origin of unlabelled skeletal elements. This paper describes the skeletal remains from Great Chesterford in terms of what has been received by the University of Southampton and provides a comparison with the original report (Waldron, 1994). Details of age, sex, preservation, completeness and pathology are included in a new inventory that has been designed as a searchable research tool in order that others may find the collection of research use. A brief discussion on the efficiency of the methods used to sort the remains is presented, in addition to the similarities and differences between the original report and the new inventory. The latter part includes the description of a number of notable pathologies absent from the original report.

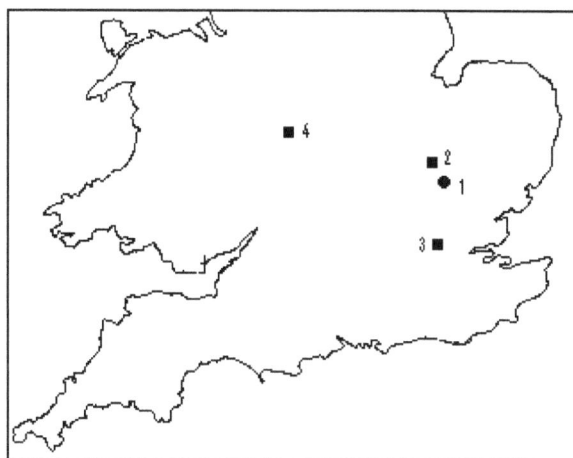

Figure 1. Location of Great Chesterford. 1: Great Chesterford, 2: Cambridge, 3: London, 4: Birmingham.

Material and methods

The material was initially sorted, as far as possible, into discrete individuals according to labels or marks upon the bones. This was carried out by Kerry Harris at the University of Southampton. Once the material was organized as far as reasonably possible, an inventory was taken following McKinley (2004). Most of the material was received in an unwashed state so all the skeletons were cleaned as much as possible using brushes. Complete washing of the remains is currently ongoing. Comparison of the new inventories, the original report and the excavation sketches highlighted which individuals appeared to have missing elements. Completeness and preservation were noted. Preservation was scored as follows (McKinley (2004) grade equivalents are in brackets):

Excellent – all cortical bone surfaces available for pathological analysis (grade 0).

Good – most cortical bone surfaces available for pathological analysis (grade 1 - 2).

Fair – some cortical surfaces available for pathological analysis (grade 3).

Poor – no cortical bone surfaces available for pathological analysis (grade 4-5).

Unfortunately, some of the skeletal elements were not labelled or the labels had become illegible over time. These remaining bones had to be sorted and assigned to individuals using macroscopic methods. A number of methods exist for sorting commingled remains, largely based on work carried out by forensic anthropologists from mass disaster, war and genocide sites (L'Abbé, 2005). Reassembly of individuals was made manageable by the existence of excavation sketches (Evison, 1994), providing basic information regarding what skeletal material was recovered at excavation. Macroscopic techniques, including taphonomic assessment and articulation were employed, including reference to the original report, metrical assessment, taphonomic damage and pathological status. It was also possible to match elements by process of elimination.

Original report

Although there was no exact catalogue of skeletal material published in the original report, excavation sketches and a brief description of the graves recorded the major elements that were present. This provided an idea of the initial completeness of the skeletons and was especially important when assigning unlabelled skulls and long bones to labelled skeletal material.

Metrical analysis

It is understood that estimates in the original report were calculated following Trotter (1970), with details of the specific elements used for each individual noted (Waldron, 1994: 59-63 App.1). Stature estimates were calculated for unassigned long bones following Trotter (1970), Trotter and Gleser (1952, 1958 and 1977). Using the same equations, estimates were recalculated for individuals that had corresponding missing elements. Stature estimates were also used to confirm the identification of long bones matched to individuals using other methods.

Pathology

Brief descriptions of pathological lesions were presented in appendix 2 of the original report (Waldron, 1994). More detailed descriptions were provided for some lesions in the main report. General information on dental, trauma, congenital, infectious, nutritional, neoplasia, degenerative and developmental conditions were provided. Descriptions of two well-healed cranial wounds were provided for individuals 101 and 75. Pathologies were used to pair up affected elements that had become separated. The presence of dental pathology was used to discriminate between individuals.

Taphonomy

On the basis of taphonomic change, some unlabelled fragmented bone could easily be matched to labelled bone fragments. For example if the proximal potion of the femur was labelled, it was usually relatively easy to match the unlabelled distal end. As grave-good staining was noted in the previous report (Waldron, 1994: 59-63), its presence was used to discriminate between elements. Consideration was given to the state of preservation and colour of the other elements of the skeleton.

Ageing and sexing

Age and sex were estimated in order to assess whether the reorganised skeleton was the same individual as stated in the excavation report. Ageing limited the number of possible individuals to which the skeletal material could belong, by restricting the possible matches to those within the correct age range. Adults were aged using the dental attrition method according to Brothwell (1994). The pubic symphyses were aged following the Suchey-Brooks methods (Suchey and Katz, 1986; Brooks and Suchey, 1990) and the auricular surfaces were aged according to Lovejoy *et al.* (1985) and Meindl and Lovejoy (1989). Where possible, age in children was estimated from dental development following Ubelaker (1989). If no teeth were present, long bones were measured and assessed. Fazekas and Kosa (1978) linear regressions were used for foetuses and full term babies, whereas infants and children were aged following the Maresh (1970) linear regression tables. The progression of epiphyseal fusion was used as an indicator of age (Scheuer and Black, 2000). Any infants equal to, or under, 36 weeks gestation were considered to be foetal: above 36 weeks gestation, infant remains were recorded as neonatal.

Sex was determined using the sexually dimorphic traits of the cranium and the pelvis. The grading of sex characteristics was as suggested by Buikstra and Ubelaker (1994), from strongly male through weakly male, indeterminate, weakly female to strongly female. No attempt was made to sex individuals below 18 years of age. Any noteworthy pathological lesions were recorded.

Results

10% of the skeletal material was either poorly labelled or unlabelled, of which approximately half could be returned to individuals. The collection still consists of 167 individuals, the same as that stated in the original report. There are, however, differences between the individuals included in new data and the original report. There is some confusion over the individual originating from grave 62; whilst the excavation plan suggests it is an adult burial (Evison, 1994:31), the bone report indicates the individual is an infant (Waldron, 1994:61). However, in the current collection, there are remains of both an adult and an infant labelled as 62. Both individuals have been included in the individual count in the current report. Two foetuses are missing from grave 83. Grave 114 now appears to contain a mixed burial of at least two individuals which were assumed to be one individual in the original report (this is discussed later). Although there were instances of unlabelled additional bones mixed with other individuals, no other new individuals were created as additional skeletal material could represent the missing elements of other known individuals. In Evison (1994: 110), grave 131 contained some excavated human bones but these now appear to be lost. This material was absent at the time of the original report and there are still no remains that can be definitely attributed to this individual.

Half of the unlabelled material could be returned to the correct grave using one or a combination of the methods described above. Table 1 displays the number of unlabelled and unassigned bones.

Table 1. Current number of unassigned bones in the Great Chesterford collection.

Skeletal element	Number
Fibulae	11
Humeri	11
Radii	5
Crania and mandibles	5
Crania	6
Mandibles	7
Femora	4
Tibiae	4
Clavicles	3
Ulnae	2
Ossa Coxae	1
Scapulae	1
Vertebrae	1

Even after sorting through the large quantity of unlabelled material, it became clear that some material from the original report is absent from the current collection. This includes the skulls of individual 75 and 101. Cranial injury 101 was consistent with a blunt force blow whereas the individual 75's injury is consistent with a sword blow (Waldron, 1994:58). Similarly, lumbar vertebrae two to five of individual 137, reported as having Pott's disease (Waldron, 1994:58), are also absent. Lesions in the currently present vertebral body of the first lumbar vertebra of individual 137 are consistent with the diagnosis of tuberculosis. No material, labelled or unlabelled, has pathology consistent with Waldron's (1994: 58) descriptions.

Stature estimates were used to return humeri to individual 22, a tall individual. Pathology was used to identify the femora of individual 152. The labelled ossa coxae of this individual had severe pitting, eburnation and remodelling in both acetabulae (Fig. 2). Two unlabelled femora were identified with corresponding lesions. There are no other femora in the collection with lesions that might correspond to those in the ossa coxae. Descriptions of caries, abscesses and antemortem tooth loss (Waldron, 1994) proved valuable for identifying mandibles, with six being returned to crania using this method. The record of dental pathology, in this case caries and antemortem tooth loss (Waldron, 1994: 63), in addition to sexing, was used to distinguish between two skulls both labelled as individual 24. The second skull remains unidentified. Extensive new periosteal bone growth on the long bones of individual 86, a juvenile of seven to nine years, indicated that an unlabelled, unfused fibula belonged to the individual.

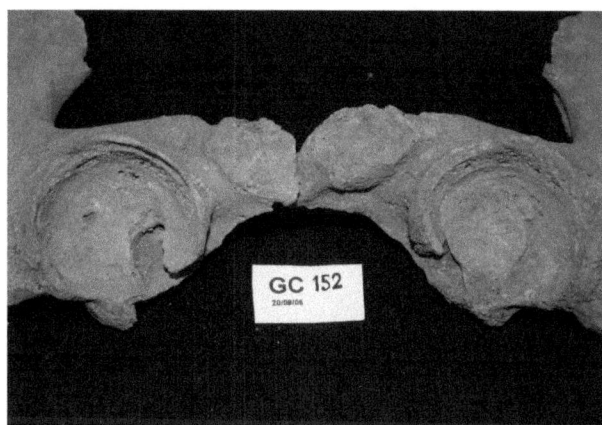

Figure 2. Eburnation, pitting and new bone growth of both acetabulae of individual 152.

Taphonomic changes provided multiple techniques for matching unlabelled skeletal material to burials. Four clavicles were labelled as belonging to individual 66, but two were eliminated as they lacked the staining arising from grave-goods described in the report (Waldron, 1994: 61). There was only one well-preserved spine (consisting of C3 – L5) that was unlabelled. Excavation damage to the anterior vertebral body of C2 of individual 103 could be aligned with the damage to the anterior vertebral bodies of the unlabelled C3 and C4. Many labelled long bones had become fragmented, unlabelled fragments were easily matched to the corresponding labelled fragment.

Taphonomic interpretation of the assemblage is affected by the missing elements. There is clear under-representation of the right foot. Considering the storage history of the collection, it is not inconceivable that the University has not received a box of right feet. It is unlikely that the absence of these skeletal elements is a result of anything other than curation and for this reason no graphic presentation of skeletal element survival has been provided in this report.

Preservation of the remains.

Preservation was scored as excellent, good, fair or poor. Table 2 displays the results of the visual analysis of the inhumations, showing the number of individuals in each preservation category. In general the preservation of the material was good.

Table 2. Visual categorisation of preservation (n.).

Excellent	Good	Fair	Poor	Total
13	103	44	7	167

Skeletal completeness

Skeletal completeness was estimated for all discrete burials. Table 3 displays the number of skeletons in each category of skeletal completeness. Twenty seven (75%) of the <25% category are juveniles. This is understandable, as due to their size and morphology, infant and juvenile bones are more likely to be lost or damaged.

Table 3. Skeletal completeness (n.).

>75%	75-50%	50-25%	<25%	Total
42	41	40	36	157 *

Demographic composition of the assemblage.

There are 167 individuals at the site. 77 are adults (M3 in occlusion and all major long bones fused), nine are sub-adult (aged 15 – 21, with some unfused bones) and 81 (15 or younger) are juvenile or infant.

Adult age and sex

Table 4 displays the data for adult age and sex at Great Chesterford. There are no significant differences between the ages in the current report and those stated in Waldron (1994). It was possible to make sex estimations for some older subadults (20, 23, 129 and 130). Individual 23 is now scored as ambiguous sex rather than female as there is disagreement between the pelvis and skull. The skull and pelvis were previously labelled and were not reunited as part of this project. There are slightly fewer females in the current report, in contrast to the findings in Waldron (1994: 52). Individuals 11, 18, 21, 26, 101, 121, 126 and 129 can no longer be sexed osteologically using the above methods, due to absent elements.

Individual 114 has a male cranium (aged 45+), an ambiguous mandible (aged 25 – 35) and ambiguous sex postcrania (auricular surface age 30 – 34 years). The difference in dental ages derived from the cranium and mandible make it clear that there are at least two individuals in the grave, not one as originally recorded (Waldron, 1994: 62). Descriptions of green staining on the mandible in Waldron (1994: 62) suggest that it was not intrusive. As this grave was disturbed and the remains

Table 4. Age and sex of the adult individuals at Great Chesterford.

Sex	M	?M	I	?F	F	Total
Young	6	3	8	6	3	26
Middle	9	4	2	8	6	29
Old	2	3	1	4	3	13
Unknown	1	-	9	2	1	13
Total	18	10	20	20	13	81

M=Male, ? M= Probably male, I= Indeterminate, ?F= Probably female, F=Female.

disarticulated, it is unsurprising that there is a mix of individuals. In addition, Waldron (1994: 62) designates this as a female grave, yet there is no clear skeletal evidence that either of the individuals are female. Although the goods associated with this grave (2 bronze small long brooches, beads and a pin (Evison 1994: 107, Table 39 164)) could be suggestive of women, researchers (Lucy, 1997:164; Stoodley, 1999: 48) have demonstrated that grave goods cannot be exclusively associated with sex. For this reason, two individuals have been included in the inventory, an old male represented by the skull, and an unknown sex middle adult, represented by the mandible. The postcrania have not been included as it could correspond to the skull or mandible.

Seventy four ear ossicles were removed from labelled crania during the process of cleaning at Southampton. These were immediately sided, bagged and stored with the associated crania from which they were removed. This would permit a small study on ear bones that are rarely found in archaeological assemblages or seldom addressed by osteoarchaeologists.

Juvenile age

There are 81 individuals aged under 15 (49%) and a further nine aged between 15 and 21 years. The high proportion of juvenile remains is worthy of attention. Thirty six individuals were aged using dental development (Table 5), sixty five using long bone measurement and seventy four using either long bone estimates or dental development (Table 6). Epiphyseal fusion was used as an age indicator. Twenty nine individuals were aged using more than one method.

Differences can be observed between long bone derived ages and dental development (Table 6), with fewer juveniles and infants aged using dental development. Foetuses and neonates are especially under-represented by dental aging in comparison to long bone age estimates. The differences between long bone and dental development sequences are discussed later. Nevertheless, the data in Table 5 highlights a good recovery of infant remains relative to other Anglo-Saxon sites. At Mucking, Essex (inhumations = 80), just five juveniles were recovered (Mays, 1992). At Butler's Field, Lechlade in

Table 5. Age categorisation of juveniles derived from dental development (Ubelaker, 1989).

Age	Individuals (n.)	Individuals (n.) in large age groupings
Birth +/- 2 months	9	9
6 months +/- 3 months	4	5
9 months +/- 3 months		
1 year +/- 4 months	1	
18 months +/- 6 months	1	3
2 years +/- 8 months	2	
3 years +/- 12 months		4
4 years +/- 12 months	4	
5 years +/- 16 months		
6 years +/- 24 months		6
7 years +/- 24 months	3	
8 years +/- 24 months	2	
9 years +/- 24 months	1	
10 year +/- 30 months		
11 years +/- 30 months	1	9
12 years +/- 36 months		
15 years +/- 36 months	8	
Total	36	36

Table 6. Age categorisation of juveniles derived from dental development (Ubelaker, 1989), long bone lengths (Maresh, 1970; Fazekas and Kosa, 1978) and both methods.

Age	Teeth	Long bones	Teeth and long bones
Foetal	0	4	4
0-2 months	9	25	29
2 months – 1 year	5	7	8
1.5 – 2 years	3	6	6
2.5 – 5 years	4	10	7
5.5 years – 10 years	6	6	8
10.5 years – 15 years	5	7	8
15.5 years – 21 years	4	-	4
Total	36	65	74

Individuals 4, 32 and 160 have lesions in the spine consistent with Pott's disease. All affected vertebrae have lytic lesions in the vertebral bodies with little or no reactive new bone growth. Individual 160 has extensive destructive lesions in the anterior vertebral bodies of T9 and T10, which have subsequently caused kyphosis of the spine (Fig. 3).

Gloucestershire, (n=198), only 33% of the inhumations were under fifteen, with just five newborns and two foetuses (Boyle *et al.*, 1998). Castledyke at Barton on Humber (n.=199) has nine children under two including six newborns (Boylston *et al.,* 1998) and just 23% of the cemetery is subadult.

Grave 83 was originally reported as containing six 36 – 40 week foetuses (Waldron 1994: 102), but in the current collection there are only four individuals represented by left tibiae. Using long bone measurements, three were aged as 38 – 40 week neonates and one as a 34 week foetus. Age estimates can no longer be calculated for individuals 56, 91, 98, 139 and 143 as they have suffered post-excavation element loss. Individual 146 can no longer be aged as two sets of teeth are labelled as GC 146 and it is difficult to tell which dentition actually belonged to the individual.

Pathology

A number of notable pathological lesions were recorded that were not addressed in the original report. It is not the purpose of this paper to present all the pathological findings, hence only a brief description of the unreported gross pathology is provided. A later paper will discuss the importance of the findings within the context of the site.

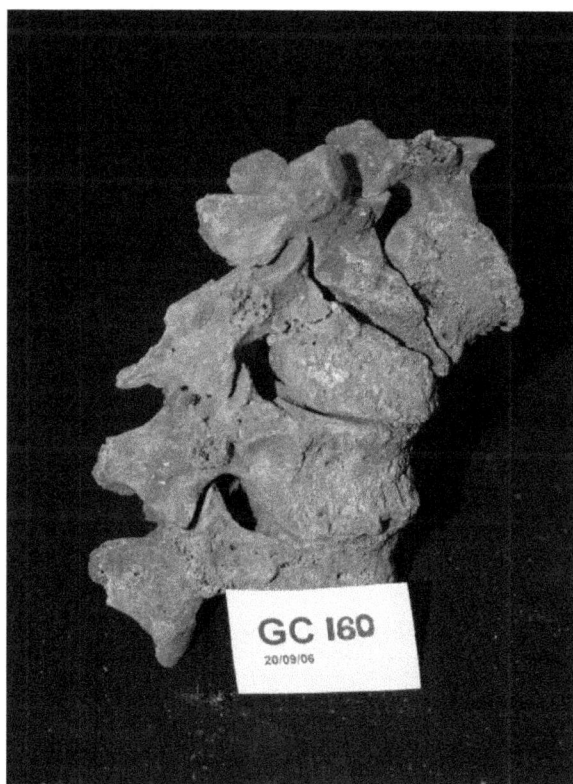

Figure 3. Individual 160. Kyphosis of the spine caused by tuberculosis.

Individual 32 has localised destruction of vertebral bodies L2 and L3. Individual 4 has lesions in T11, T12, L1, L2 and the inferior of T2, in addition to destruction between the left sacral foramina one and two. Unlike tuberculosis, osteomyelitis of the spine does not spare the vertebral arches, facets or spinous processes (Ortner, 2003). Similarly, the lack of reactive new bone formation is indicative of tuberculosis, rather than osteomyelitis. A differential diagnosis of brucellosis is being considered for individual 4, who exhibited a multi-focal infection with some involvement of a superior articular facet (Fig. 4). Although destruction was extensive in some vertebrae, they did not collapse. Brucellosis infection begins in the intervertebral disc space but can lead to osteomyelitis (Glasgow, 1976).

Individual 128, a young male adult, has extensive destruction of the left acetabulum and complete destruction of the left femoral head (Fig. 5). Limited signs of infection suggest that the loss of the femoral head was traumatic. This may have been caused by trauma that cut off the blood supply to the unfused femoral head epiphysis subsequently causing necrosis of the femoral head (Knüsel pers comm.). However, the extensive damage caused to the femoral neck is unusual of trauma and the smooth surface of the proximal femur may be more indicative of tuberculosis. Manchester (pers comm.) describes femoral head and neck destruction in more advanced hip tuberculosis. The destruction of the acetabular floor is particularly characteristic of tuberculosis (Manchester pers comm.). New bone growth limited to the visceral surface of the ribs is another

Individual 96, a young male, has active and remodelled periostitis on the distal thirds of both tibiae and fibulae. The new bone is orientated longitudinally but takes on a nodular appearance where the new bone is thickest, particularly along the interosseous borders. There are also destructive lesions to the feet (Fig. 6). The second, third and fifth right metatarsals have mid-shaft pencilling and almost complete destruction to the distal articular surfaces. Thick periostitis surrounds the mid-shaft of the left first metatarsal and portions of the left second metatarsal. The head of the right first metatarsal and the proximal joint surface of the corresponding hallical phalange have osteitis. The combination of pencilling of the metatarsals, destruction to the tarsals and periostitis of the distal third of the tibiae and fibulae are indicative of leprosy (Aufderheide and Rodríguez-Martín, 1998). The cranium is too damaged for assessment of facies leprosa.

Three juveniles (34, 86 and 106) have substantial new bone growth distributed throughout the skeleton, particularly focused on long bone diaphyses. The lesions have striking symmetry between the left and right sides. All three have visceral rib lesions. There are a few possible causes of this, including infantile scurvy and hypertrophic osteoarthropathy. One characteristic of scurvy is subperiosteal bone deposition on long bones. However in scorbutic infants subperiosteal haemorrhage is normally limited to the metaphysis and only reaches the diaphysis in extreme cases (Aufderheide and Rodríguez-Martín, 1998: 311). Porosity of the greater wing of the sphenoid, the orbital roof, maxilla and occipital is a characteristic of scurvy in infancy and childhood (Ortner and Ericksen, 1997). No abnormal cranial porosity was identified in the three individuals. It seems unlikely that scurvy would be the cause of the diaphyseal lesions.

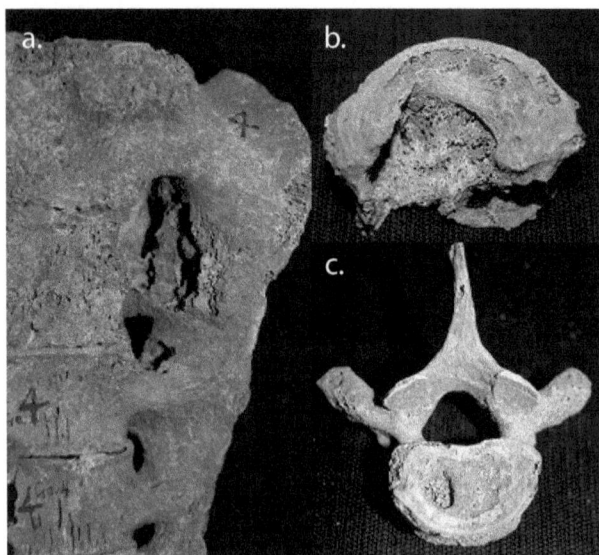

Figure 4. Individual 4, a) destructive lesion in S2/S1, also note new bone growth on the anterior surface of the sacrum, b) multiple lytic lesions in L1, c) lesion on inferior aspect of body of T2.

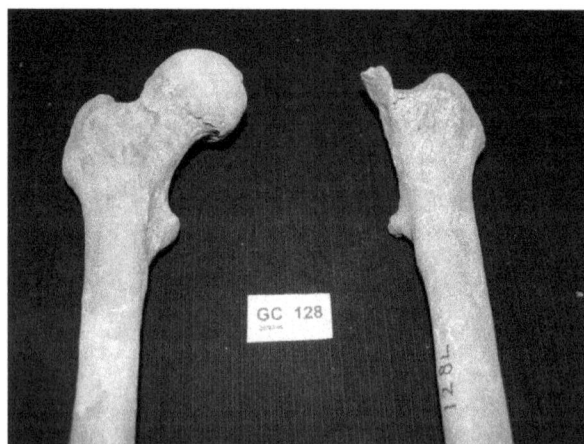

Figure 5. Individual 128. Destructive lesions to the left femoral head and neck.

indicator of tuberculosis (Santos and Roberts, 2006) and was visible on the ribs of individual 128. This individual also suffers from mild osteoarthritis in the lower spine, possibly linked to the subsequent superior dislocation of the femur.

Hypertrophic (pulmonary) osteoarthropathy (HPO) produces symmetrical lesions distributed throughout the skeleton, particularly focussed on the subperiosteal surfaces of long bone diaphysis and are often linked to intra-abdominal or intra-thoracic disorders (Mays and Taylor, 2002) including tuberculosis and other respiratory diseases. The visceral rib lesions suggest a pulmonary infection, potentially tuberculosis. However limited clinical documentation of HPO diagnosed in young individuals in the literature makes this diagnosis problematic, especially in the case of individual 34 (one year old). Further analysis is required on these individuals. Finally, individual 152 has severe bilateral osteoarthritis of the hips. The new bone growth and eburnation on the joint surfaces are features that are associated with osteoarthritis (Ortner, 2003).

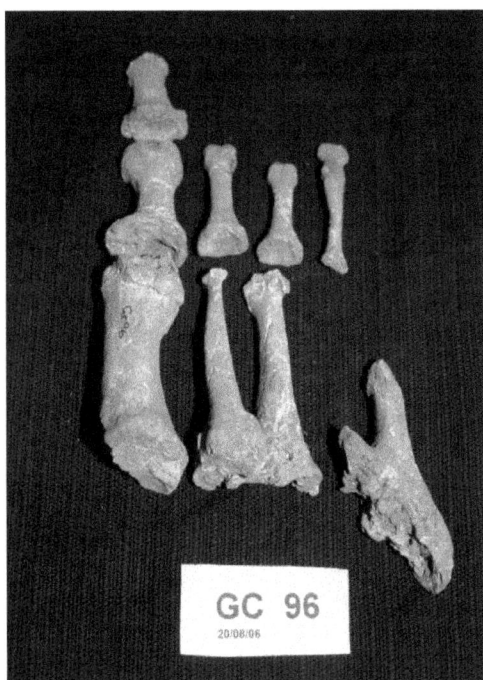

Figure 6. Individual 96. Pencilling of second, third and fifth metatarsals with destructive lesions to the proximal joint surfaces possibly caused by leprosy.

Discussion

Inadequate storage of the Great Chesterford skeletal material has caused damage to the collection. It is also apparent that not all of the skeletal material has been received by the University of Southampton. It is often the case that pathological specimens are selectively removed for incorporation in museum or teaching collections. Although the 50% of unknown skeletal material could be returned to the correct individual using one or a combination of methods described above, methodological limitations means some skeletal material cannot be returned to the correct individual. The methods employed rely on gross morphological techniques, including matching through pathology, taphonomy, articulation, and the process of elimination (L'Abbé, 2005). These matching methods are only useful when there is something unique or infrequent about a bone or skeleton. For example, replacing elements for individuals with tall or short stature estimates was straightforward but problematic for individuals within the average height range.

Articulation was constructive for matching crania to postcrania, as the atlas and axis were frequently stored with the skull, whereas the rest of the spine remained with the postcrania. The closer the fit between particular elements, the more successful articulation was. For example, L'Abbé, (2005) considers the low level of fit between the scapula and humerus to be the reason why there are often more unidentified humeri than femora in a sample under study. This is also the case with the Great Chesterford collection, where 11 humeri remain unidentified compared with just four femora (Table 1). The presence of pathology was only useful when severe or of a rare condition. The process of elimination often limited the possible matches, but when there were large numbers of unlabelled elements it was impossible to make a decision with a reasonable level of certainty.

Once all the material was sorted into discrete individuals, there were few discrepancies between the current age, sex and number of individuals in comparison to the original report (Waldron, 1994) (except individuals 23 and 114). Differences occurred where individuals can no longer be aged or sexed using the above methods. This is especially true for individuals 18, 21, 26, 126 and 129 who were all initially recorded as female (Waldron, 1994) but are now unsexed. These individuals account for the higher quantity of females in the original report.

Three methods were used to obtain the maximum possible information on age from the juvenile individuals (dental development, long bone linear regression and epiphyseal closure). Comparison of the long bone and dental age estimates (Table 6) indicates a difference between the mortality profiles. Tooth development sequences indicate far fewer neonates and infants than suggested from the long bone lengths. This is caused by the loss of such small teeth during excavation or curation. However, as teeth tend to preserve better than other human material, when bone preservation was insufficient for the measurement of the long bones, tooth development could still be analysed. Table 5 has been created with wide age estimates to present a more inclusive mortality profile. However, it was sometimes unclear which age category some individuals fell into as the long bones always had a lower age estimate than indicated by dental development. Furthermore, with increasing age, the disparity becomes larger. In some cases (individuals 23, 21, 36 and 79) the long bone age estimate failed to reach the lowest possible tooth development age. For example individual 23, is dentally aged adult because the M3s have erupted and exhibit some occlusal wear, thereby suggesting an approximate age of 21. However, all the major long bones are unfused proximally and distally. In addition, the glenoid fossa and coracoid of the scapula are also still unfused. It would be expected that both the proximal and distal epiphyses of all the long bones would be fused by age 18 if female and 20 if male.

There are a number of possible reasons for the disparity between the ages calculated from long bones and tooth development. First, the applicability of the methods to this particular population needs to be considered. Both sets of ageing standards have been compiled from modern living individuals or those of known age at death, thus their application to the Great Chesterford population may be problematic. In fact, Hoppa (1992) found that the Anglo-Saxon children analysed in his sample had the smallest rates of growth and by early adolescence the difference between the modern and Anglo-Saxon individuals could be as much as four years (Hoppa, 1992). The Great Chesterford individuals follow the trend of smaller children for age. White and Folkens (2005) suggest that if long bone lengths are used for the estimation of age, a close comparison population is required, which, unfortunately for most archaeological populations, is not usually available. Nutritional and health care improvements have probably led to the increase in growth rates in modern individuals and comparison to these are likely to under-age archaeological populations (Mays, 1999).

Second, studies have demonstrated that nutritional stress can delay epiphyseal fusion, increasing the growing period (Mays, 1999). It is considered that dental development is less affected by environmental factors than skeletal growth (Ubelaker, 1989). Even in children living around the poverty line, dental emergence is only slightly delayed and, in fact inter-population variation appeared to create more variation (Garn *et al.*, 1973). The above reasons could explain why a number of individuals have unfused proximal and distal long bones but adult dentition with some M3 occlusal wear. Although hypoplasia and cribra orbitalia may be additional evidence for nutritional stress within the Great Chesterford population, the level of severity is minor and there are no obvious cases of scurvy or rickets. In addition individuals who had no pathological lesions were also under-aged. It therefore seems less likely that the individuals have been affected by malnutrition.

Through detailed examination of the material, it became apparent that some of the bones required more attention than was initially given in the original report. Some of the bones, when cleaned, had pathological lesions that had not been originally described. One such example was individual 4, where mud in the vertebrae obscured cavitation. In addition to individual 4, the author and Dr Simon Mays identified three further possible cases of tuberculosis (individuals 32, 128 and 160). A number of other individuals (22, 34, 86, 106) have visceral rib lesions and other non-specific new bone growth that may be related to a chronic pulmonary infection. Great Chesterford was previously considered to have a low level of infectious disease however this recent assessment shows this is not the case. These pathologies are of importance and further work is being carried out to assess the significance of the pathologies within the context of the site.

The high recovery of child remains is unusual for Anglo-Saxon sites, yet reflects the quantity of infant and juveniles that would be expected of the Anglo-Saxon period. Often preservation at early Anglo-Saxon sites is fair to poor and it is postulated that infant and juvenile remains fail to survive in hostile soil conditions (Buckberry, 2000). However, preservation is complex and remains are found unexpectedly in poorer soil environments (Buckberry, 2000). This insinuates that other factors play a role in the low level of infant and juvenile remains, including shallower burials, burial away from the rest of the population or differential disposal. In this respect, Great Chesterford is a distinctive site.

Conclusions

Great Chesterford highlights the plight of many human skeletal collections where inadequate labelling (which is considered obligatory in lithics and ceramics) is still not yet mandatory in archiving human skeletal remains. Sorting the skeletal remains from Great Chesterford has taken over a year to complete, with the vast majority of time being taken by trying to sort out and organise unlabelled elements. 50% of the unlabelled remains were returned to the correct individuals through the use of the original report and macroscopic methods. Unfortunately, some of the skeletal material will remain unidentified as it is uncertain to which burial the element originated. This is largely due to the limitations of the methodologies, which fail to differentiate between average individuals or elements that have no distinct characteristics.

The catalogue can be used as a research tool, containing data on age, sex, preservation, completeness and other useful traits and pathologies. The data can be easily searched to ascertain whether the collection would be suitable for any research needs. It is intended that additional data will be added to the inventory in the future in order to aid other researchers.

The high level of juvenile recovery is an interesting feature of the site. In addition, the unreported cases of tuberculosis and other pathological material will be of interest to other researchers. Despite a few missing elements and some unlabelled material, the collection still can be used for research into social and economic aspects of Anglo-Saxon England.

Acknowledgements

Many thanks are due to Dr. Sonia Zakrzewski of the University of Southampton for granting access to the Great Chesterford collection. Dr Simon Mays is thanked for his thoughts on pathologies. Dr. Jo Sofaer, Dr. Sonia Zakrzewski, Kris Poole and Katey Edwards kindly commented on drafts of this paper. Emma Pomeroy and Amanda Di-Loreto are thanked for their unpublished data on age and sexing.

Literature cited

Aufderheide, A. and Rodríguez-Martín, C. 1998. *The Cambridge Encyclopedia of Human Paleopathology.* Cambridge: Cambridge University Press.

Boyle, A., Jennings, D., Miles, D. and Palmer, S. 1998. *The Anglo-Saxon cemetery at Butler's Field, Lechlade, Gloucestershire.* Volume 1: Prehistoric and Roman activity and Anglo-Saxon grave catalogue. Oxford: Thames Valley Landscapes Monograph number 10, Oxford Archaeology Unit.

Boylston, A., Wiggins, R. and Roberts, C. 1998. "Human skeletal remains" In: Drinkall, G. and Foreman, M.A. *The Anglo-Saxon Cemetery at Castledyke South, Barton-on-Humber.* Sheffield: Sheffield Academic Press. 221-236.

Brooks, S.T. and Suchey, J.M. 1990. "Skeletal age determination based on the os pubis: a comparison of the Acsádi-Nemeskéri and Suchey-Brooks methods" *Human Evolution* 5:227-238.

Brothwell, D.R. 1994. *Digging Up Bones.* 3rd ed. London: Oxford University Press.

Buckberry, J. 2000. Missing, presumed buried? Bone diagenesis and the under representation of Anglo-Saxon children. http://www.assemblage.group.shef.ac.uk/5/buckberr.html. Date accessed 10/05/07.

Buikstra, J.E. and Ubelaker, D.H. 1994. *Standards for Data Collection from Human Skeletal Remains.* Fayetteville: Arkansas Archaeological Survey.

Evison, V. 1994. *An Anglo-Saxon Cemetery at Great Chesterford, Essex.* York: Council for British Archaeology Research Report 91.

Fazekas, I.G. and Kosa, F. 1978 *Forensic Fetal Osteology.* Budapest: Akadémiai Kiadó.

Garn, S.M., Nagy, G.M., Sandusky, S.T. and Trowbridge, F. 1973. "Economic impact on tooth emergence" *American Journal of Physical Anthropology* 39:233-238.

Glasgow, M.M.S. 1976. "Brucellosis of the spine" *British Journal of Surgery* 63:283-288.

Hoppa, R.D. 1992. "Evaluating human skeletal growth: an Anglo-Saxon example" *International Journal of Osteoarchaeology* 2:275-288.

L'Abbé, E.N. 2005. "A case of commingled remains from rural South Africa" *Forensic Science International* 151:201-206.

Lovejoy, C.O., Meindl, R.S., Pryzbeck, T.R. and Mensforth, R.P. 1985. "Chronological metamorphosis of the auricular surface of the ilium: A new method for the determination of at death" *American Journal of Physical Anthropology* 68:47-56.

Lucy, S.J. 1997. "Housewives, warriors and slaves? sex and gender in Anglo-Saxon burials." In: Moore, J. and Scott, E. (eds.) *Invisible People and Processes. Writing Gender and Childhood into European Archaeology.* London: Leicester University Press. 150-168.

Maresh, M.M. 1970. "Measurements from roentgenograms". In: McCammon, R.W. (ed.) *Human Growth and Development.* Charles C Thomas: Springfield, Illinois. 157-200.

Mays, S.A. 1992. Anglo-Saxon human remains from Mucking, Essex. Ancient Monument Laboratory Report 39/93. Unpublished report, English Heritage.

Mays, S.A. 1999. *The Archaeology of Human Bones.* London: Routledge.

Mays, S.A. and Taylor, G.M. 2002. "Osteological and biomolecular study of two possible cases of hypertrophic osteoarthropathy from mediaeval England" *Journal of Archaeological Science* 29:1267-1276.

McKinley, J.I. 2004. "Compiling a skeletal inventory: disarticulated and commingled remains". In: Brickley, M. and McKinley, J.I. (eds.) *Guidelines to the standards of recording human remains.* Institute of Field Archaeologists 7. 14-17.

Meindl, R.S. and Lovejoy, C.O. 1989. "Age changes in the pelvis: Implications for paleodemography". In: Iscan, M.Y. (ed.) *Age Markers in the Human Skeleton.* Charles C Thomas: Springfield, Illinois. 137-168.

Ortner, D.J. 2003. *Identification of Pathological Conditions in Human Skeletal Remains.* London: Academic Press.

Ortner, D.J. and Ericksen, M.F. 1997. "Bone changes in the human skull probably resulting from scurvy in infancy or childhood" *International Journal of Osteoarchaeology* 7:212-220.

Santos, A.L. and Roberts, C.A. 2006. "Anatomy of a serial killer: Differential diagnosis of tuberculosis based on rib lesions of adult individuals from the Coimbra identified skeletal collection, Portugal" *American Journal of Physical Anthropology* 130:38-49.

Scheuer, L. and Black, S. 2000. *Developmental Juvenile Osteology.* London: Academic Press.

Stoodley, N. 1999. *The Spindle and the Spear.* Oxford: British Archaeological Reports, British Series 288.

Suchey, J. and Katz, D. 1986. "Skeletal age standards derived from an extensive multiracial sample of modern Americans" *American Journal of Physical Anthropology* 69:269.

Trotter, M. 1970. "Estimation of stature from intact limb bones". In: Stuart, T.D. (ed.) *Personal identification in mass disasters.* Washington. National Museum of Natural History. 71-84.

Trotter, M. and Gleser, G.C. 1952. "Estimation of stature from long bones of American Whites and Negroes" *American Journal of Physical Anthropology* 10: 463-514.

Trotter, M. and Gleser, G.C. 1958. "A re-evaluation of estimation of stature based on measurements of stature taken during life and of long bone after death" *American Journal of Physical Anthropology* 16:79-123.

Trotter, M. and Gleser, G.C. 1977. Corrigenda: "Estimation of stature from long limb bones of American whites and negroes" *American Journal of Physical Anthropology* 47: 355-356.

Ubelaker, D.H. 1989. *Human skeletal remains*. Second Edition. Washington: Taraxacum Press.

Waldron, T. 1994. "The human remains". In: Evison, V. (ed.) *An Anglo-Saxon Cemetery at Great Chesterford, Essex.* York: Council for British Archaeology Research Report 91. 52 – 66.

White, T.D. and Folkens, P.A. 2005. *The Human Bone Manual*. London: Academic Press.

Rickets in Victorian London: why treatment was ineffective for so long

Lisa Brent[1] and Piers D. Mitchell[2]*

[1]Imperial College London School of Medicine, [2]Faculty of Medicine Imperial College London
*e-mail address for correspondence: piers.mitchell@imperial.ac.uk

Abstract

This research aims to investigate the medical treatment of rickets in London during the 1800s, using the techniques of both palaeopathology and medical history. Study of skeletal changes to selected long bones and crania held in the pathology collection at Imperial College London was undertaken. The marked bowing of lower limbs and cranial vault changes demonstrated that there were severe cases of Vitamin D deficiency. These findings raised the question as to how the Victorians, renowned for their major scientific advances, failed to prevent a condition so easy to treat as rickets. Publications on rickets dating from the 1800s were then studied. It was found that in the early nineteenth century humoural imbalance was the dominant theory, following the work of Glisson from 1651. By the second half of the 1800s, descriptions of the condition were becoming more accurate, and in 1883 Barlow differentiated the symptoms of rickets alone from rickets combined with scurvy. It was only by the mid 1880s that cod liver oil (high in vitamin D) was commonly prescribed to those that could afford medical advice. In 1890 Palm proposed lack of sunlight to be the main underlying cause of the condition, as we now know to be the case. For decades the Victorians failed to appreciate the consequences of childhood factory labour, atmospheric smog and housing design upon sun exposure. Despite the Victorian advances in medical technology, hygiene and microbiology, they remained largely powerless against the simplest of diseases in their own capital city, namely rickets.

Keywords: rickets, Victorian Period, London, cod liver oil, scurvy

Introduction

As the capital of the British Empire, Victorian London was renowned for the great scientific discoveries announced there. Technologies such as microscopes, x-rays, and anaesthetics were enabling pioneering medical research (Snow, 2006:2) and general mortality rates were decreasing (Hardy, 1992:389-391). However, rickets (Vitamin D deficiency in children) remained a major cause of deformity and disability to thousands living in this capital. This research investigates how such a situation arose and offers an explanation as to why.

Examples of skeletal evidence will be examined for rickets dating from 1800s London. The changing perceptions of the Victorian medical community to rickets are then investigated. The varying ideas and aetiological theories that were explored, together with their influence on treatments for rickets are then summarised. Finally, there is discussion and conclusion as to why rickets was so common in the late nineteenth century, forty years after an effective treatment had been found.

Aetiology of rickets

Rickets is a disease of infancy and childhood, typically developing from the age of four months to two years (Ortner, 2003:393). It is characterised by an excess of unmineralized osteoid matrix due to insufficient Vitamin D (Smith and Wordsworth, 2005:173) which occurs whilst the skeleton is still growing (Whyte and Thakker, 2005:70). When Vitamin D deficiency occurs after the epiphyses have fused (i.e. in adults) it is termed osteomalacia (Whyte and Thakker, 2005:70). Rickets is most commonly caused by lack of sunlight, rather than by dietary deficiency (Molleson and Cox, 1993:45; Mays, 2003:144). This is because the primary human source of vitamin D is produced in the skin, as cholecalciferol, by the photoactivation of 7-dehydrocholesterol (Mays, 2003: 144; Reginato and Coquia, 2003:166). Rickets can also be caused by chronic renal tubular failure, a lack of calcium and phosphorous in the diet, chronic liver and intestinal disorders, hereditary defects and drugs (Reginato and Coquia, 2003:1064). In rickets the changes in the growing bone are complicated by inadequate provisional calcification of the epiphyseal cartilage, thus causing the derangement of endochondral bone growth of long bones (Rauch, 2003:75). The result is deformation of the skeleton due to the loss of structural rigidity of the developing bones (Smith and Wordsworth, 2005:175). Short stature can also result due to physeal disturbances (Whyte and Thakker, 2005:70). These changes can be observed in skeletal remains from the past allowing diagnosis by palaeopathologists. The more obvious deformities such as bowing of the legs and bossing of the skull can also be noted during life, and would have allowed a clinical diagnosis to be made by Victorian medical practitioners.

Skeletal manifestations of rickets

The skeletal manifestations depend on the severity of the rachitic process, its duration and in particular, the stresses to which individual bones are subjected. They are described here to more comprehensively understand the skeletal examples and the extracts from Victorian medical texts presented. As a non-ambulatory infant, the head and chest are subject to the greatest stresses (Kumar *et al.*, 2005:454). The rapidly growing and expanding cranial vault of the infant with rickets is increasingly replaced by non-mineralized osteoid, as a part of the remodelling of the infant skull to accommodate the growing brain. This gives rise to areas of thinning and softening, 'craniotabes' (Ortner, 2003:396). Craniotabes may lead to a permanent posterior flattening, or, lateral and asymmetrical deformities of the skull due to pressure of the head against the supporting surface in the supine position. Closure of the fontanelles is also delayed in rickets. During the process of remodelling, the outer and often inner table disappears so that the entire thickness of the cranial vault has the porous appearance of diploe and can resemble the bone changes seen in chronic anaemia (Ortner, 2003:394). An excess of osteoid can produce bossing of the frontal and parietal bones (Smith and Wordsworth, 2005:177). In regard to chest deformities, the 'rachitic rosary' consists of prominent beads resulting from overgrowth of cartilaginous osteoid tissue at the costochondral junction of ribs. The weakened metaphyseal areas of the ribs are subject to the pull of the respiratory muscles and so bend inwards, creating an anterior protrusion of the sternum (pigeon breast deformity/ pectus carinatum) (Kumar *et al.*, 2005:455).

When an ambulating child develops rickets, deformities are likely to affect the spine, pelvis and long bones, causing most notably a lumbar hyperlordosis and bowing of the legs (Kumar *et al,.* 2005:455). Particularly characteristic changes include; broadening ('flaring') and 'cupping' of the metaphyseal areas of long bones (Ortner, 2003:394). These changes represent the variations found in the width of the osteoid borders of rachitic long bones. The amount of uncalcified bone matrix usually parallels the degree of change at the metaphyseal epiphyseal junction (Follis, 1958:374). When the deformities develop in the active phase, a compensatory alteration of the subperiosteal bone occurs, resulting in increased deposition on the concavity of the deformity in response to the altered stresses. If adequate vitamin D later becomes available, osteoid formed during active rickets will mineralize (Ortner, 2003:396) and healing will take place (Follis, 1958:378). The healing process involves the deposition of inorganic materials in the matrix adjacent to the most recently matured chondrocytes. The mineralization process then spreads to involve portions of the rest of the cartilage. However, much of the hypertrophic region is never calcified and is eventually destroyed by osteolysis (Follis, 1958:378). With healing (i.e. when the affected individuals are no longer vitamin D deficient) major deformities become long standing and are followed by characteristic remodelling changes. The curved bones show a decreased transverse and an increased anteroposterior diameter. There is complete alteration of the trabecular pattern with new trabeculae crossing the medullary cavity in a radial arrangement, converging to the concavity of the curve (Ortner, 2003:397).

Although none of the following features identified are diagnostic on their own, in combination they enable the recognition of rickets in skeletal material for active disease in immature remains (Mays *et al.*, 2006:363). The osteoarchaeological criteria defined by Ortner and Mays (1998:46) and relevant to this project include: cranial vault porosity, deformed lower limb bones, long bone changes (metaphyseal flaring, general thickening, metaphyseal porosity, concave curvature porosity), superior flattening of the femoral metaphysis, *coxa vara* and porosis of bone underlying long bone growth plates. Radiographic criteria (Mays *et al.*, 2006:369) consist of trabecular coarsening/thinning, loss of cortico-medullary distinction, cortical tunnelling and alteration of biomechanical architecture.

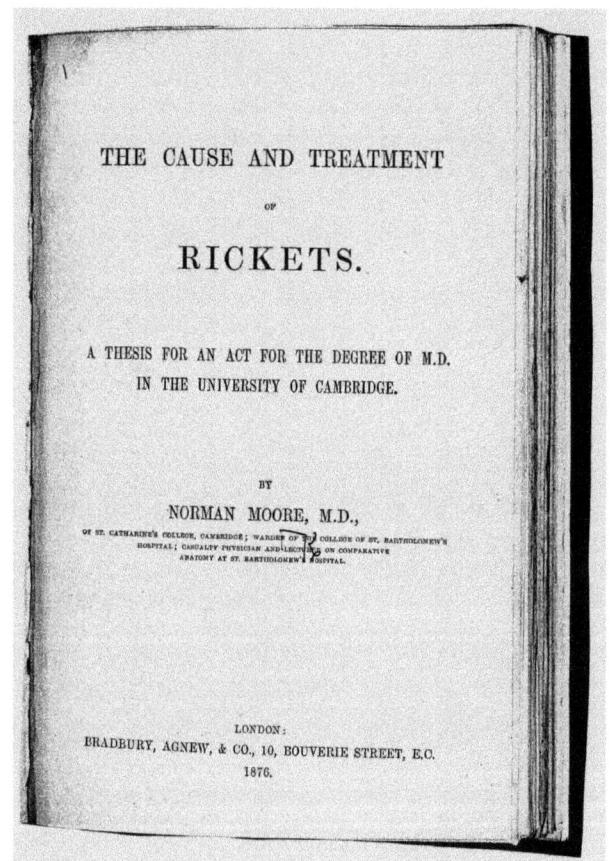

Figure 1. Book title page from Moore's thesis on rickets, dating from 1876.

Materials and methods

Skeletal examples of rickets dating from the 1800s were examined in combination with textual evidence from the Victorian era (1837-1901). Two specimens of skeletal material from the Imperial College London hospital pathology museum were examined (codes 1503 and 1507). These specimens were originally obtained by the Westminster Hospital pathology collection, London, which was later amalgamated with the Imperial College collection. The material in the Westminster pathology collection was mostly derived from post mortem examinations of the London poor. The museum catalogue cards show that these two specimens were obtained prior to 1900. Macroscopic and radiographic changes from the skeletal material were noted in order to confirm the diagnosis, and also to enable a better understanding of the pathological descriptions in the Victorian textual sources.

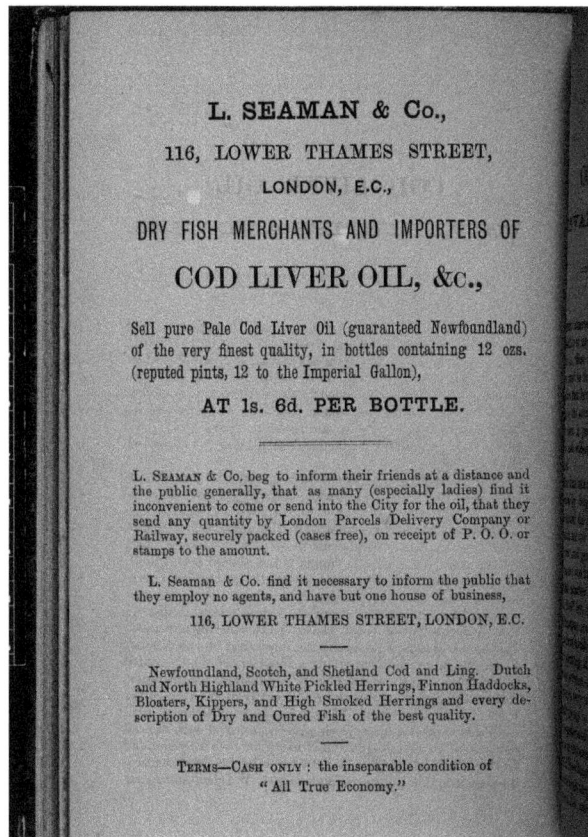

L. SEAMAN & Co.,

116, LOWER THAMES STREET,

LONDON, E.C.,

DRY FISH MERCHANTS AND IMPORTERS OF

COD LIVER OIL, &c.,

Sell pure Pale Cod Liver Oil (guaranteed Newfoundland) of the very finest quality, in bottles containing 12 ozs. (reputed pints, 12 to the Imperial Gallon),

AT 1s. 6d. PER BOTTLE.

L. SEAMAN & Co. beg to inform their friends at a distance and the public generally, that as many (especially ladies) find it inconvenient to come or send into the City for the oil, that they send any quantity by London Parcels Delivery Company or Railway, securely packed (cases free), on receipt of P. O. O. or stamps to the amount.

L. Seaman & Co. find it necessary to inform the public that they employ no agents, and have but one house of business,

116, LOWER THAMES STREET, LONDON, E.C.

Newfoundland, Scotch, and Shetland Cod and Ling. Dutch and North Highland White Pickled Herrings, Finnon Haddocks, Bloaters, Kippers, and High Smoked Herrings and every description of Dry and Cured Fish of the best quality.

TERMS—CASH ONLY : the inseparable condition of "All True Economy."

Figure 2. Advertisment for cod liver oil, © The British Library. (shelfmark 7461.aaa.74) All Rights Reserved.

Texts written by the medical profession dating from the 1800s were studied. In order to understand the knowledge base inherited by the Victorians, earlier texts were consulted that recorded the beliefs of clinicians in the mid-seventeenth century, when the first printed works on rickets were published. After a discussion of these ideas, the major ideas and publications throughout the Victorian period, regarding the understanding of the pathophysiology of the disease, its identification, treatment and prevention will be analysed. Medical journals studied include the Edinburgh Medical Journal, The Lancet and the British Medical Journal. The articles are a combination of individual case reports, pathology papers, essays, clinical lectures and theses (Fig. 1). Some of these sources were written by men held in very high esteem during this time, such as Sir Thomas Barlow, and are frequently used by modern authors when writing about historical perspectives of rickets. The work of other, less well known authors has also been analysed including that of Chance (1862) Godlee (1884) Jenner (1895) Moore (1884) Railton (1894) Ransom (1899) and Stephenson (1865). These sources explore the views of the medical profession about rickets clinically, pathologically and therapeutically. In addition, texts by analytical chemists and advertisements from pharmaceutical companies (Fig. 2) were studied to help

reveal how medical advances regarding the treatment of rickets were filtering down to the public.

Results

Skeletal material

Macroscopic pathological changes were documented using Ortner and Mays' criteria for active infantile rickets (Ortner and Mays, 1998: 46). Radiographic changes were documented using palaeopathological (Mays, *et al.* 2006: 369) and clinical (Murray and Jacobson, 1977: 657) criteria. The pathology specimens were in a good state of preservation. However, a limitation was that the entire skeleton for each case was not preserved, just the individual bones with the most notable pathology. In consequence, the overall skeletal distribution pattern in this disease could not be determined.

Specimen 1503 was a set of four abnormal long bones, with no clear evidence as to whether they were from the same or separate individuals (Figs. 3 and 4). No further skeletal material relating to these specimens was available. There were two femora, a tibia and its corresponding fibula. Each was from an adult individual displaying evidence of healed rickets from childhood. All the bones demonstrated bowing which was most pronounced in the middle third of the shaft. There was also flattening of the shaft to give an oval cross section, and buttressing with supplementary bone on the concave aspect. The proximal and distal joint surfaces were no longer parallel as a consequence of the bowing, and this is best appreciated in the case of the tibia and fibula. A rachitic deformity such as bowed legs affects both the appearance and gait of an individual (Molleson and Cox, 1993: 26) so walking with the sole of the foot on the floor would undoubtedly have been difficult for this individual. One femur also demonstrated coxa vara with a neck-shaft angle reduced to 90 degrees, in contrast to the normal angle of approximately 130 degrees.

A key differential to exclude is the possibility that specimen 1503 is simply an incomplete set of bones with osteomalacia or healed osteomalacia. In osteomalacia the principle defect is of remodelling, not modelling (Whyte and Thakker, 2005: 70). This is because the epiphyses have fused and modelling changes have essentially ceased. This means osteomalacia is not usually deforming (unless fractures occur) and impaired skeletal mineralization is much less apparent clinically and radiographically (Whyte and Thakker, 2005: 70). This is in stark contrast to the gross deformities shown by specimen 1503. It is unlikely that the individuals were vitamin D deficient when they died. Many remodelling changes have taken place in an attempt to reinforce the rickety bones which could not have occurred with unmineralized, vitamin D deficient bone. For example, evidence of buttressing with deposition of dense, ivory like-bone on the concave aspect (best seen on the femur in cross section) is an attempt to reinforce the rickety femur. A similar phenomenon occurs with the trabeculations

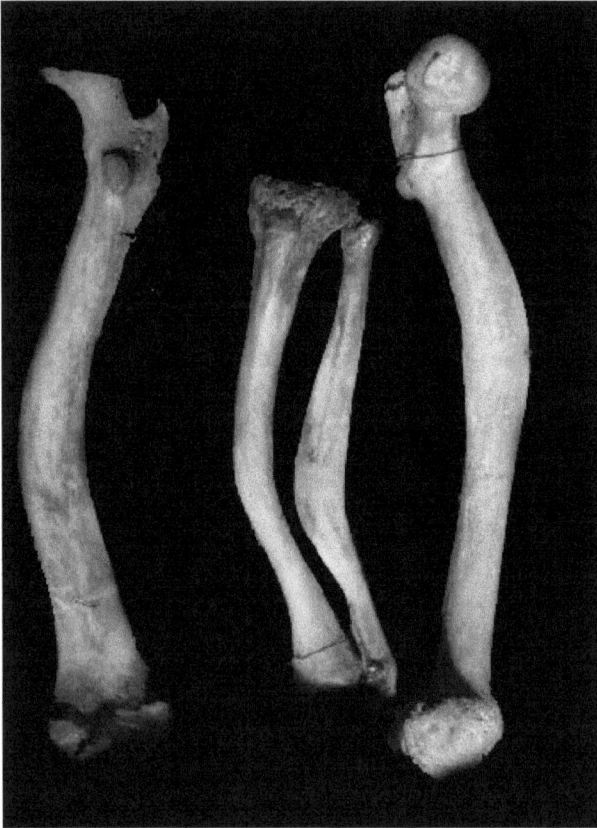

Figure 3. Specimen 1503, dating from the Victorian Period. Femora, tibia and fibula demonstrating deformed lower limb bones, and metaphyseal flaring. The femur on the right also has *coxa vara* (not visible on this view).

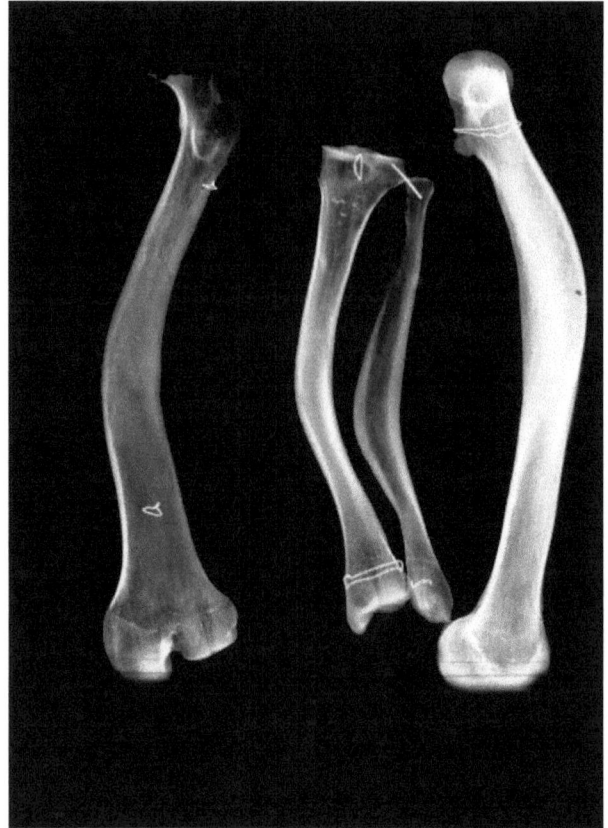

Figure 4. Specimen 1503, radiograph demonstrating trabecular coarsening/ thinning, loss of cortico-medullary distinction, and biomechanical alterations.

of cancellous bone. The previously radially arranged trabeculations (consistent with healing changes in rickets, Ortner, 2003: 397) have become longitudinally arranged at the diaphysis in an attempt to distribute the weight more evenly. Finally, another probable indicator that these bones were from adult individuals with healed rickets and no longer vitamin D deficient at the time of death, is the presence of abnormal Harris lines on the superior metaphysis of the tibia (Figs. 3 and 4). Harris lines are dense, opaque, transverse lines representing periods of stress when growth in length has been arrested. Suggested causes include nutritional deficiencies or childhood disease (Roberts and Manchester, 2005: 240). Harris lines can only occur when the bones are growing but can be detected at all ages (Grolleau-Raoux *et al.*,1997:210). They are effectively, 'recovery lines' as they can only occur when the individual has recovered from the stress episode (Roberts and Manchester, 2005:240). A person continually malnourished and diseased will not display Harris lines (Roberts and Manchester, 2005:240) These are defective Harris lines because each individual line does not extend fifty percent or more across the bone shaft. This could be because the lines were being remodelled away due to continual bone turnover as the individual aged and had partially resorbed at the time of the individual's death (Grolleau-Raoux, *et al.*, 1997:210; Roberts, 2005:240-241).

Specimen 1507 was a calvarium of a child approximately under the age of two years, as the anterior fontanelle had not closed by the time of death (Figs. 5 and 6). On macroscopic inspection it was noted to be asymmetrical, with right frontal and left parietal bones enlarged compared with the contralateral sides. The dimensions from right frontal to left parietal were 15.3cm, compared with 13.9cm for left frontal to right parietal. Parietal bossing was also visible on the anteroposterior view. There is diffuse porosity of much of the outer table and this was most marked at the parietal and frontal eminences. The internal aspect of the calvarium demonstrates craniotabes, a feature of both infantile scurvy and rickets. The spongy diploe of the bone was virtually absent around the majority of the circumference of the skull, being less than 1mm thick. The bone is so thin that on careful macroscopic inspection the imprint of the cerebral convolutions can be seen, and this is even clearer on plain radiographs (Fig. 6). There were only three areas where the diploe was thicker, measuring approximately 3mm. The first area was at the region of the frontal crest. The other two were bilateral lesions, one stretching approximately 5cm on the left side, and one approximately 3cm on the right side. Both lesions are situated so that they correspond to where the *temporalis* muscle of mastication lies. In previous papers (Ortner and Ericksen, 1997:212, 213; Brickley and Ives, 2006:164) this sign has been linked as being evidence of scurvy, as the weakened and defective blood vessels resulting from vitamin C deficiency are more susceptible to damage

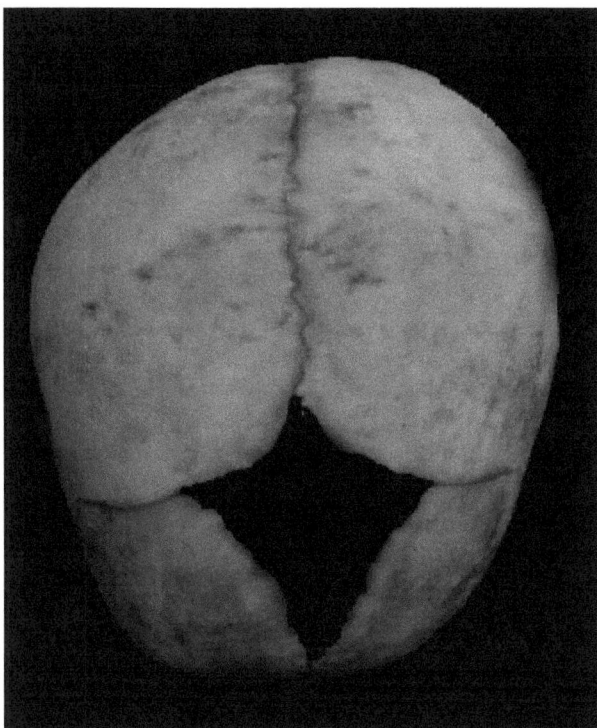

Figure 5. Specimen 1507, dating from the Victorian Period. Cranium demonstrating signs of scurvy-rickets. This view best shows the asymmetry, due to deficient mineralization of the developing skull.

during chewing. Chronic haemorrhaging from the deep vasculature associated with the temporalis muscle would explain the porosity in these regions. In consequence, this specimen probably displays evidence of both rickets and scurvy and this will be discussed later in the context of 'scurvy-rickets'.

Textual sources

Francis Glisson and seven other doctors of 'physick' and Fellows of the College of Physicians of London wrote the treatise *De Rachitide* over five years (Glisson, 1650; Moore, 1884:71). This was originally published in Latin in 1650, and again in English in 1651. The treatise was an influential piece of work "justly regarded as one of the monuments of English medicine" (Moore, 1884:71) and is one example of the views of the medical profession at this time. These doctors believed that rickets was a new and fatal disease (Glisson, 1651:8). The majority of the treatise focuses on the aetiology of rickets, which was centred upon beliefs regarding one's constitution, spirits, the balance of their humours and the six non-naturals. Until 1800, medical theory was essentially based on 'learned medicine', which relied on the ideas and practices of the ancient Greeks, mainly humoralism, constitution and temperament. The system of regimen involved maintaining humoral balance appropriate to temperament and centred on the six non-naturals (respiration, food and drink, exercise and rest, sleep and waking, expulsion and retention of fluids and affections of the mind). The humoral theory was easily understood

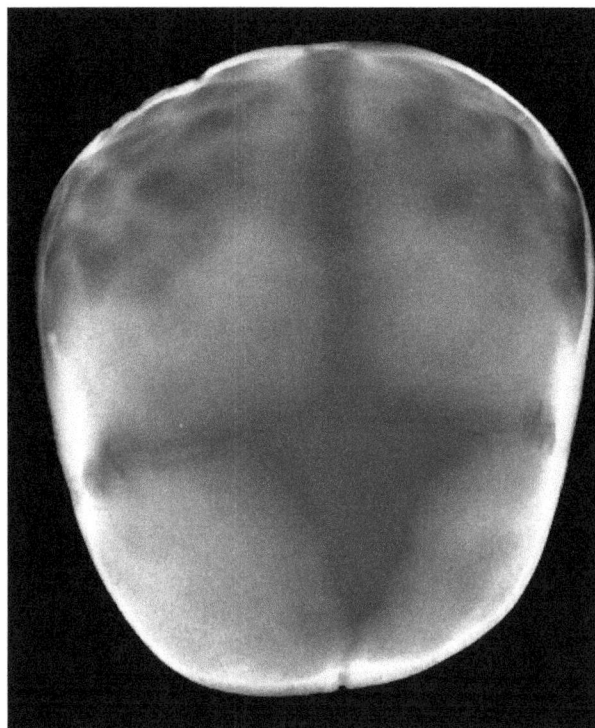

Figure 6. Specimen 1507, radiograph highlighting indentation by the cerebral convolutions.

and often used by the public (Wear, 1987:235). Glisson *et al.* concluded that "the essence of this disease (rickets) consists...in the natural constitution" (Glisson, 1651:26) and that the area of the body responsible for causing the disease was "the special marrow issuing out of the skull" (Glisson, 1651:54).

In terms of identifying the disease there were endless signs and symptoms for most body parts. It is clear that both the understanding of the disease and the diagnostic criteria in use were very different from those accepted today (Whyte and Thakker, 2005:70) (Table 1). However, there are certain features described, some of which are mentioned in the following excerpts from the original text, which do comprise the key clinical signs of rickets as it is defined today: 'The top of the ribs to which the stern (sternum) is conjoined with gristles, are knotty like unto the joints of the wrist and ankles' (Glisson, 1651:12) "The Stern is somewhat pointed like the keel of a ship or the breast of a hen" (Glisson, 1651:12). "They whose thigh and shank bones are much increased, rather according to the latitude and thickness, then according to longitude, for the most part become dwarfs" (Glisson, 1651:256). These features describe very well the characteristic rachitic deformities we would now term the rachitic rosary, widened epiphyses, *pectus carinatum*, and bowing of the legs, respectively. The doctors held the belief that these bony changes marked the 'continuence' of the disease (Glisson, 1651:252). It was believed by Glisson and his colleagues that this disease primarily affected the rich, "the cradles of the gentry" (Glisson, 1651:252). It was believed that being middle class "those privileged by a mediocrity of fortune" (Glisson, 1651:252), helped to prevent this disposition.

In terms of treatment, 'the best nourishment' (Glisson, 1651:290) and topically and internally administered medicines were advised. Nourishment was advocated because it was believed the extra bone of the swollen areas "requireth a fuller nourishment" (Glisson, 1651:291). In addition to typical treatments of humoural medicine such as purging, the use of leeches and bloodletting, (Glisson, 1651:252) "artificial erection" of the crooked bones was recommended (Glisson, 1651:291) "not only for strength but also to correct the crookedness of the bones" (Glisson, 1651:318). A detailed account of how to make one's own splints was given, including labelled pictures giving a step-by-step guide (Glisson, 1651:318-320). In terms of prognosis, factors giving a worse outcome included the extent of "crookedness" (of certain bones) and of "the inflexion of the joints" (Glisson, 1651:253, 254). If the child had not been cured before reaching the age of five, it was suggested that the child would either die at an earlier age than other children with rickets or they would "grow deformed, crooked and dwarfish" (Glisson, 1651:256).

The Victorian Period was more proliferative in terms of the amount of literature produced, so there are a greater variety of opinions expressed in a number of sources. Dr Stephenson described "a characteristic history of rickets" where symptoms were listed as "diarrhoea, great restlessness, crying, thirst, heat of skin and refusal of food" (Stephenson, 1865:613). Stephenson acknowledged that though a child with rickets may not show every symptom, there are certain symptoms which are to be regarded as "specially diagnostic of the disease" (Stephenson 1865:614). These symptoms include the child sleeping with a great disinclination to being covered; the child perspiring greatly about the head when they slept; the face being flushed during sleep and pain in response to touch (Stephenson 1865:612-614). Stephenson did however acknowledge that in regard to having these specially diagnostic symptoms, "some medical men…doubt the accuracy of this opinion" and believed that these symptoms also occurred in other constitutional diseases (Stephenson, 1865:614).

Many of these symptoms would appear to have nothing to do with rickets as we know it today, with the exception of "pain in response to touch" possibly representing bone pain which can be found in rickets (Whyte and Thakker, 2005:70) or scurvy (Weinstein *et al.,* 2001:57). However, when noting the observational findings of the child he wrote:

"Head of moderate size; anterior fontanelle large; bones otherwise firm. There is a distinct enlargement of the bones at the wrist; legs straight; slight lateral compression of chest; sternum and cartilages prominent and rounded throughout the whole extent" (Stephenson, 1865:613).

The diagnostic signs that he looked for to identify the disease are similar (but incomplete) to what a modern clinician would seek to identify today. However, it appears that no uniform set of diagnostic criteria had been established across the medical profession by the time this article was written in 1865. One example of this diagnostic discontinuity is when Stephenson commented that he differed from other writers "who state craniotabes or soft occiput to be 'very common' " (Stephenson, 1865:615). This line indicates there was not a united opinion for craniotabes and soft occiput being two clinical manifestations of rickets.

In terms of aetiology the profession believed that the 'exciting cause' or precipitating cause was induced by dentition (teething) but that the primary cause of the disease was the rachitic constitution (Stephenson 1865:613). Stephenson's belief was that although a parent who had suffered from the disease could not pass on rickets to their child, children could inherit a tendency predisposing them to the rachitic constitution from the "morbid tendency of the constitution derived from the mother" (Stephenson, 1865:616). Stephenson also discusses the reasoning for his belief in the rachitic constitution as opposed to the popular idea that rickets was caused by poor hygiene:

"Writers on this subject have endeavoured to account for the origin of rickets by the multitudinous anti-hygienic influences to which children are subject; but the fact that all children, alike exposed, do not become rachitic, has led to the belief in a constitutional predisposition" (Stephenson, 1865: 616).

The level of aetiological misunderstanding is again highlighted when Stephenson remarks that if "bone affection alone (were) to be taken as the mark of disease" then doctors might misdiagnose the condition as tuberculosis instead of rickets (Stephenson, 1865:615).

Dr. Cheadle described rickets in the terms of its bony manifestations, including enlargement of the ends of long bones and beading of the ribs, but also "laboured and stridulous" breathing (Cheadle, 1878:685). *Laryngismus stridulous* was a term used to describe this difficult breathing. In the context of a symptom of rickets this was later redefined to a supervention of bronchitis/pneumonia when the child was profoundly cachexic, which could then cause death (Moore, 1876:13; Barlow, 1894:1075). Rickets was still regarded as a fatal disease (Barlow, 1883:176; Jenner, 1895:5). Rickets was also mentioned by many authors as being a scrofulous disease (Bell, 1834:918; Smythe, 1844:21) although there was some debate about this (Bennett, 1841a:101; Chance, 1862:184; Jenner, 1895:8). Jenner recognised rickets and tuberculosis as two separate diseases (Jenner, 1895:8). He gave a mostly accurate description of the disease, including the histology, where he described a defect in chondrocyte calcification of the matrix (Jenner, 1895:12-13). He even commented on malnutrition, although he also admitted that this was a very vague term (Jenner, 1895:8). There is no reference to sunlight despite Palm's paper of 1890 describing its relationship to rickets:

Table 1. A comparison of the modern and historical criteria of rickets.

Modern criteria for rickets	Historical criteria for rickets
Age: 4 months - 2years[1] Aetiology: Vitamin D deficiency (or resistance)[2] Clinical Features: Bone pain/tenderness Muscle weakness (myopathy) Signs of tetany from associated hypocalcaemia Pathological fractures in the diaphyses of long bones[2] Skeletal deformity: Delayed closure of fontanelles, bossing of frontal and parietal bones,[1] craniotabes, bowing of the long bones, swollen epiphyses, beading of the ribs (rachitic rosary), short stature[2], pectus carinatum, Harrison's sulcus, deformities of pelvis and spine (lumbar hyperlordosis), frontal bossing[3] Radiology: AP view of knees and PA view of wrists show widening of growth plates, Metaphyseal splaying, Cupping of epiphyses[2]	**Pre-Victorian**[1] Age: infant – 5 years + Aetiology: natural constitution, the special marrow issuing out of the skull. Affects 'cradles of the gentry' Clinical Features: Fatal, irregularity and disproportion of body parts, slender and extenuated external membranes and muscles of the whole body, hanging skin, protuberant abdomen, large liver, flatulent tumours of stomach and gut, ulcers etc. Skeletal deformity: rachitic rosary, swollen epiphyses, pectus carinatum, bowing of the long bones, short stature, tumours of bone **Victorian** Aetiologies: Primary cause = constitutional disease due to morbid tendency of the mother Exciting cause = induced by dentition/teething Poor hygiene[2] Decreased breastfeeding, increased use of proprietary foods, rickety diet[3] Clinical Features: Diarrhoea, great restlessness, crying, thirst, heat of skin, refusal of food, weakness, pale, dull complexion, cachexia, sweating, delayed teething, sleeping with a great disinclination to be covered, perspiring greatly about the head during sleep, facial flushing during sleep, pain in response to touch[2], Laryngismus stridulous[4], fatal[5], tooth decay, pectus carinatum, short stature, feeble pulse, delay in walking, aversion to being shaken, cough[6], scrofulous (debated) Skeletal Deformity: Bones do not have to be affected, delayed closure of fontanelles, soft bones, swollen epiphyses, bowing of the legs, large angular head, rachitic rosary, lateral chest compression, craniotabes and soft occiput (debated)[2]
[1] Ortner 2003:393-396 [2] Whyte and Thakker 2005:70 [3] Kumar *et al.* 2005:455	[1] Glisson 1651:12-252 [2] Stephenson 1865:613-616 [3] Barlow 1894:1076-1079 [4] Cheadle, 1878:685 [5] Barlow 1883:176 [6] Moore 1876:10

"a deficiency of (sunlight) characterises the localities or conditions of those who suffer from rickets, and this is the most important element in the aetiology of the disease" (Palm, 1890: 274).

Jenner noted that weight bearing combined with softened bones caused the curvatures of long bones (Jenner, 1895:14-16). He also described the rachitic deformity we today call Harrison's sulcus (Jenner, 1895:16). However, he mentioned that many well esteemed pathologists still believed rickets, scrofula and tuberculosis were the same disease, whilst others suggested rickets was a variety of congenital syphilis (Jenner, 1895:8). The idea of congenital syphilis was generally seen as a differential diagnosis and is mentioned in numerous case reports as a relevant negative in the context of the rachitic history (Cheadle, 1882:48; Barlow, 1883:161,191; Godlee, 1884:60; Railton, 1894:532). Exclusion of syphilis was based on the history of the child's parents, particularly the mother (Barlow, 1883:194).

In the last quarter of the nineteenth century there was still reference to rickets being a constitutional disease (Moore, 1876:34; Jenner, 1895:4). However, it seems that the profession started to gradually replace the term "constitution" with "condition" (Cheadle, 1878:687), perhaps representing the phasing out of the humoural theory. The medical profession believed that a decreased breastfeeding rate amongst mothers (Moore, 1876:31, 35; Barlow, 1894:1079), and the "enormous increase…in the employment of proprietary infant foods" were underlying causes of the disease process (Barlow, 1894:1079; Ransom, 1899:1257).

The treatments delivered by the medical profession were described by Stephenson as "cod-liver oil, iron and improving hygienic conditions" (Stephenson, 1865:619). Cod-liver oil contains high concentrations of vitamin D, however, the profession at this time had not identified vitamin D as a distinct chemical substrate, and were simply offering cod-liver oil as a treatment because of previous experience (Stephenson, 1865:619).

In 1878 Dr Cheadle wrote a paper outlining the idea that scurvy and rickets was occurring simultaneously in some children, (Cheadle, 1878:685,686) with scurvy supervening upon rickets (Cheadle, 1878:685,687). Much of the pathophysiology of scurvy given in the Victorian literature was correct and described features such as, blood vessel fragility and swollen gums (Cheadle, 1878:685). Defective osteoid formation, fragile blood vessels and their resultant haemorrhages are still seen as skeletal hallmarks of scurvy today (Kumar *et al,.* 2005:458,459; Brickley and Ives 2006:163) and such skeletal manifestations are visible on the calvarium examined as part of this study. Cheadle believed scurvy was caused by "a scurvy diet" (Cheadle, 1878:686). Similarly, he believed that a "rickety diet", which consisted mainly of farinaceous (wheat based) food, caused rickets "with the greatest regularity and certainty" (Cheadle, 1878:687). Cheadle mentioned that rickets was the most common complaint at the Children's Hospital (Great Ormond Street) but that scurvy was extremely rare in comparison. He attributed a lack of potatoes in the diet as the reason to why these children with rickets also suffered from scurvy (Cheadle, 1878:687). The deficiencies in both Vitamin C and D simultaneously would perhaps today be reasoned by general dietary deficiency or malnourishment. Dietary deficiency is more likely to cause a deficiency in several vitamins than a deficiency in a single vitamin alone (Kumar, *et al.* 2005:450).

Barlow endorsed Cheadle's work (Barlow, 1894:1076) and published an extensive review of the issue in 1883, which he then updated in 1894. Both doctors believed fresh foods (Cheadle, 1878:686), or 'living foods' (Barlow 1894:1078), were the correct treatment. They came to this conclusion by noting the patient's condition at presentation and then again after the diet was changed accordingly. Marked improvements were often seen as little as three days later (Cheadle, 1878:686). However, there was some confusion between the true aetiology and

treatment for each disease. For example, Barlow (1894: 1078) believed that "fresh air and sunshine" aided recovery of scurvy-rickets after implementing dietary changes but that they would not prevent the onset of the disease. Barlow never advocated exposure to sunlight for rickets alone, where the greatest therapeutic benefit would have been gained.

By 1884 doctors were prescribing cod liver oil (Moore, 1876:33) and lemon or orange juice to treat the condition of "scurvy-rickets" (Godlee, 1884:61; Railton, 1894:532). These are now known to be among the richest dietary sources of vitamins D and C respectively. Although 'vitamins C and D' had not yet been discovered, the cause and treatment of scurvy and diet induced rickets had essentially been discovered.

Far from being a new medicine, cod-liver oil was used around the world as a popular remedy for rheumatic diseases for over a century (Bennett, 1841a:13; Bennett, 1841b:215; Horsley, 1856:5; Willmott, 1860:91). It was also used to treat "rachitis" (Bennett, 1841b:215). In 1771, cod-liver oil attracted the limited attention of the medical profession in England (Willmott, 1860:91) although dates vary (Bennett, 1841a:14,15; Souther, 1849:4; Horsley, 1856:5). Dr Bennett is accredited with introducing it to the wider notice of the medical profession in England in 1841 (Willmott, 1860:93; Seaman, 1869:5)[1] However, it was a long time before cod-liver oil actually came into general use in England, the chief reasons being the "disgusting character (taste) of the oil" and the "very questionable process by which it was prepared" (Willmott, 1860:91). Willmott believed that if it were not for the many successes of the Germans with this remedy, it would have been employed "little, if at all" as a treatment in England (Willmott, 1860:91). The pale and light brown varieties were used medicinally (Willmott, 1860:96) in a number of conditions including rickets (Willmott, 1860:119). In 1841, Dr. Bennett believed cod-liver oil to be a "general roborant" (Bennett, 1841b:215) and that the most marked benefit for this remedy was in "genuine rachitis and scrofulous disease" (Bennett, 1841b:216). He believed that it was not successful in every case but that it had the advantage of not causing harm (Bennett, 1841b:217). It seems to have been primarily used for pulmonary consumption according to later sources (Willmott, 1860:120; Seaman, 1869:5). Willmott believed that many diseases originated in "one and the same cause" so it was rational for "one and the same remedy" to cure them all (Willmott, 1860:119). Many theories as to the mechanism of action were proposed, but the most common idea was that it was a "dietetic article of easy assimilation" (Willmott, 1860:110). It was believed that cod-liver oil's fattening properties were due to the fact that it caused the return of one's appetite (Chapman 1849:8; Horsley, 1856:10). Cod-liver oil was both internally administered and externally applied (Willmott, 1860:120) and "imperfectly nourished infants" were given 2-3 spoonfuls/day

---

[1] L.Seaman & Co. were a pharmaceutical company and in this case the written source is an informative advertisement.

(Bennett, 1841a:61; Seaman, 1869:10). Reports were given by many doctors agreeing with the use of this remedy, although there was still dissent. One doctor, Dr James Alderson, remarked that a true physician would not use this "vaunted specific" to cure people and that those who did were "pretenders and quacks" (Willmott, 1860:134).

Cod-liver oil was described as being used to successfully treat rickets (Souther, 1849:4) when all other remedies have failed or when children seemed to be on their death-beds (Chapman, 1849:8). Seaman and colleagues reported that many poor were prevented from using cod-liver oil because of the "factitiously high price at which it is usually sold" (Seaman, 1869:15). Dr. Bennett believed that the reason why cod-liver oil was so scarcely known as a remedy by the medical profession was because it was "a favourite with some empirics" (Bennett, 1841b:217). In consequence, some of the medical profession may have shunned it as they tried to distinguish themselves from lesser-educated providers of health care.

Discussion

In the early 19th century physicians believed that rickets was caused by the humoural imbalance of one's constitution. As the decades passed the diagnosis was confused by the myriad of other symptoms attributed to rickets. Infections in children often present clinically in a very non-specific way, for example, being feverish and irritable with poor feeding and sleeping habits. These symptoms were not caused by rickets itself but by other diseases simultaneously developed by the vulnerable child with rickets. Rickets plays a role in lowering a child's resistance to diarrhoeal, respiratory and tubercular infections, which makes this suggestion even more likely (Hardy, 1992:391). Some infections, such as scarlet fever (Hardy, 1992:392; Molleson and Cox, 1993:184-185), diphtheria, croup, measles and whooping cough were fatal (Hardy, 1992:392). In the 1890s, death rates for children aged between one and five were 24.3 per thousand and for infants under the age of one, were 181.2 per thousand, the main contributor for infant deaths being diarrhoeal infections (Hardy, 1992:389,390). Rickets itself is not a fatal disease and it is normal for children to survive it with an associated longstanding skeletal deformity (for example, the adult individuals with healed rickets represented by specimen 1503 in this project). It is therefore one possibility that deaths caused from supervening infection were mistakenly attributed to rickets, hence the belief by many contemporary authors that rickets was a fatal disease.

Throughout the Victorian period several references are made to the symptom of stridor/ *laryngismus stridulus* (Stephenson, 1865:619; Barlow 1883:175). This symptom can be caused by hypocalcaemia in severe rickets (Pettifor, 2005:41; Smith and Wordsworth, 2005:178). Hypocalcaemia refers to serum calcium/ calcium levels in the blood lower than the normal range, which is 2.1 – 2.5 mmol/litre (Murphy and Williams, 2005:55). It can be an asymptomatic biochemical finding,

mildly symptomatic (paraesthesia/ tingling) or severely symptomatic. Severe levels of hypocalcaemia (<1.9mmol/litre) are required to produce symptoms such as cardiac arrhythmias (Murphy and Williams, 2005:57) and stridor. However, the symptom of stridor may have been more likely to arise due to a complicating secondary respiratory infection, or when in conjunction with night sweats and weight loss, a tubercular infection, rather than rickets. Perhaps this is why many authors commented on rickets in the context of scrofulous disease.

There were no universally agreed criteria for the identification of rickets in the Victorian period. Due to differing opinions and diagnostic confusion, rickets would have been greatly misdiagnosed. The majority of the misdiagnoses were probably due to the over-diagnosis of rickets, with many additional irrelevant symptoms attributed to rickets. However, it is also clear that if doctors such as Stephenson were dismissing signs, such as craniotabes/ soft occiput, then some cases of rickets were also being missed.

Another seemingly contradictory theme is that of the relationship of rickets and social class. Glisson remarked that rickets affected the children of wealthy families, "the cradles of the gentry", whilst children from the middle class were relatively spared of this fate (Glisson, 1651:252). Authors from the Victorian period believed rickets was a disease of the poor (Stephenson, 1865:612; Barlow, 1894:1079; Jenner,: 1895:9). Barlow believed that "although the children of the poor are rickety, they are much less frequently scorbutic than the children of the rich" (Barlow, 1894:1079). Barlow's reasoning for this was because of decreased breast feeding and increased use of proprietary foods in the children of the rich (which the poor could not afford to buy). He wrote that even when the poor used condensed milk, they gave their children mixed diets (including the powerful anti-scorbutic, potatoes) at a much earlier age than the rich parents did. Jenner wrote that rickets was "by no means limited to the poor, or to London, or to large towns" and that he had often seen rickets in children of wealthy parents in the countryside (Jenner, 1895:9). It is tempting to conclude that the main cause of rickets in children of the rich, living in the countryside was diet induced, whereas children of the poor, living in cities, acquired rickets due to the pollution of the city and long hours spent toiling in factories or being brought up inside workhouses. However, this is not the case. Cheadle wrote about cases of scurvy-rickets affecting both rich and poor in London (Cheadle, 1878:685). Rickets was present in all social classes (Hardy, 1992:391; Molleson and Cox, 1993:45) but was largely an urban disease due to the smoke produced from industry and domestic heating, building practices that excluded sunlight from houses and social practices (Hardy, 1992:391,398). In terms of children of the poor, the indoor lifestyle of factories and workhouses had a detrimental effect on sunlight exposure. However, their cramped housing conditions meant that children were encouraged to go outside (Hardy, 1992:400). Concepts of respectability meant that children of the respectable poor were often in worse condition than the very poor. The respectable poor often kept their children indoors "for fear that they should mix with the 'little street Arabs' and get into bad habits" (Hardy, 1992:398,406). However, the smothering social practices of the rich (Knecht-van Eekelen and Maat, 1986:23) meant that children of wealthy families also suffered from rickets. Precautionary measures were taken by the rich to prevent contagion entering the nursery, for example, keeping the child in a room which was sealed as far as possible to exclude ventilation (Dick, 1922:419, 420).

The writings of Victorian authors have shown this was a time when hypotheses and ideas were being formulated and investigated to try and determine the cause of rickets. The irony is that during this time some expressed the opinion that rickets was a neglected disease because much histopathological investigation but little clinical work was taking place (Stephenson, 1865:613). Ideas regarding the identification of the disease, its aetiology and treatment were not accurate. It was only in 1890 Dr Palm deduced that rickets was caused by lack of exposure to sunlight and only in 1919 that Dr Huldschinsky proved this experimentally (Gibbs, 1994:731). Originally rickets was seen as a disease of the wealthy but as the frequency of the disease rose (reaching peak prevalence in the late nineteenth and early twentieth century) it was clear the greatest prevalence was amongst the poor (Mays, 2003:148,149). The differential expression of the disease amongst varying social classes at different time periods affected the theories of aetiology of the disease and ultimately how to treat it. The Victorians were unaware that sunlight deprivation was the major cause of rickets and therefore missed the most effective treatment – exposure to sunlight. Many factors including the London smog, social and dietary practices of more affluent families and the indoor lifestyle of poor children toiling in factories or workhouses had a significant aetiological role. However, the presence of both scurvy and rickets simultaneously in a minority of children suggests that malnutrition played an aetiological role in some cases.

The treatments delivered included fish oil, which was prescribed for rickets as early as the 1840s. However, its high price meant that the majority of affected children, the London poor, did not receive it until the 1880s. Cod-liver oil is a rich source of vitamin D and can be used successfully in many cases. However, as mentioned previously, it is the action of sunlight on a pro-hormone in our skin that is the primary source of vitamin D in humans. The ideal treatment was not being offered to those suffering from rickets because the true aetiology was not known.

Conclusion

Rickets seems to have been a major problem in the industrial cities of Britain in the 1800s. This is highlighted by the marked examples held in the Imperial College London pathology museum. In the 1600s the medical profession believed the underlying cause to be humoural imbalance. However, scientific research during the 1800s resulted in this theory being discarded. Victorian doctors encountered many difficulties whilst attending to patients with rickets, not least the difficulty in distinguishing which symptoms were due to rickets and which were from other conditions commonly afflicting the poor. It was probably this diagnostic confusion, combined with the high price of fish oil and doctors' reluctance to prescribe it out of professional pride, that delayed the effective treatment of rickets prior to the 1880s in London.

Acknowledgements

Dr. Dominic Blunt kindly carried out the radiography at Charing Cross Hospital, London

Literature cited

Barlow, T. Sir. 1883. "On cases described as 'Acute Rickets' which are probably a combination of scurvy and rickets, the scurvy being an essential, and the rickets being a variable element" *Medico-Chirurgical Transactions* 66: 159-219.

Barlow, T. Sir. 1894. "The Bradshaw Lecture on infantile scurvy and its relation to rickets". *The Lancet* 144: 1076-1080.

Bell, C. Sir. 1834. "Anatomy and Physiology. Lectures illustrated by the Hunterian preparations" *The Lancet* 21: 912-919.

Bennett, J.H. 1841a. *A Treatise on the Oleum Jecoris, Arseli or Cod-liver Oil as a Therapeutic Agent in Certain Forms of Gout, Rheumatism and Scrofula; with Cases.* Edinburgh: Maclachlan, Stewart and Co.

Bennett, J.H. 1841b. On the medicinal properties of fish liver oil" *The Medico-Chirurgical Review and Journal of Practical Medicine* (New Series), 36: 215-217.

Brickley, M. and Ives, R. 2006. "Skeletal manifestations of infantile scurvy" *American Journal of Physical Anthropology* 129: 163-172.

Chance, E.J. 1862. "*On the nature, causes, variety and treatment of bodily deformities. In a series of lectures delivered at the City Orthopaedic Hospital in 1852.* London: T.T Lemare.

Chapman, H.T. 1849. *On the use of cod-liver oil in diseases of the bones and joints, in consumption and in other maladies attended by great emaciation.* London: J and I Tirebuck.

Cheadle, W.B. 1878. "Clinical lecture on three cases of scurvy supervening on rickets in young children" *The Lancet* 112: 685-687.

Cheadle, W. B. 1882. "Osteal or periosteal cachexia and scurvy" *The Lancet* 120: 48-49.

Dick, J.L. 1922. *Rickets*. London: William Heineman.

Follis, R.H. 1958. *Deficiency Disease*. Illinois: Charles C. Thomas.

Gibbs, D. 1994. "Rickets and the crippled child: an historical perspective" *Journal of the Royal Society of Medicine* 87: 731.

Glisson, F. 1650. *De Rachitide*. London: George Bate and Abasuerus Regemorter.

Glisson, F. 1651 *Treatise of the Rickets: Being a Disease so Common to Children*. Translated by P. Armin. London: Peter Cole in Leaden-Hall.

Godlee, R.J. 1884. 'A case of so called scurvy rickets'. *The Lancet* 123: 60-61.

Grolleau-Raoux, J.L., Crubézy, E., Rougé, D., Brugne, J.F. and Saunders, S.R. 1997. "Harris Lines: A study of age-associated bias in counting and interpretation" *American Journal of Physical Anthropology* 103: 209-217.

Hardy, A. 1992. "Rickets and the rest: Child-care, diet and the infectious children's diseases, 1850-1914" *The Society for the Social History of Medicine* 5: 389-412.

Horsley, J. 1856. *Medicated cod-liver oil, historically and chymically considered with some account of several new methods of importing it to greater medicinal efficacy*. London: John Churchill.

Jenner, W. 1895. *Clinical lectures and essays on rickets, tuberculosis, abdominal tumours and other subjects*. London: Rivington, Percival and Co.

Knecht-van Eekelen, A. and Maat, G.J.R. 1986. Rickets and Osteomalacia. *Organorama* 23: 23-25.

Kumar, V., Abbas, A.K. and Faustro, N. (eds.) (2005) *Robbins and Cotran Pathologic basis of disease Seventh Edition*. Pennsylvania: Elsevier Saunders. 452-459.

Mays, S. 2003. "The rise and fall of rickets in England". In: Murphy, P. and Wiltshire, P.E.J. (eds.) *The Environmental Archaeology of Industry*. Oxford: Oxbow. 144-153.

Mays, S., Brickley, M. and Ives, R. 2006. "Skeletal manifestation of rickets in infants and young children in a historic population from England" *American Journal of Physical Anthropology* 129: 362-374.

Molleson, T. and Cox, M. 1993. *The Spitalfields Project. Volume 2: The Anthropology. The Middling Sort*. Council for British Archaeology Research Report Number 86. York: Council for British Archaeology. 45–215.

Moore, N. 1876. "The cause and treatment of rickets" In: *Medical Tracts 1876-1877*. London: Bradbury, Agnew and Co. 5-35.

Moore, N. 1884. "The history of the first treatise on rickets" *Saint Bartholomew's Hospital Reports* 20: 71-82.

Murphy, E. and Williams, G.R. 2005. "Hypocalcaemia" *Medicine* 33: 12:55-57.

Murray, R.O. and Jacobson, H.G. 1977. *The Radiology of Skeletal Disorders*. Second Edition, Volume 1. London: Churchill Livingstone. 652-665.

Ortner, D.J. 2003. *Identification of Pathological Conditions in Human Skeletal Remains*. Second Edition, London: Academic Press.

Ortner, D.J. and Ericksen, M.F. 1997. "Bone changes in the human skull probably resulting from scurvy in infancy and childhood" *International Journal of Osteoarchaeology* 7: 212-220.

Ortner, D.J. and Mays, S. 1998. 'Dry-bone manifestations of rickets in infancy and early childhood'. *International Journal of Osteoarcheaology* 8: 44-55.

Palm, T.A. 1890. "The geographical distribution and aetiology of rickets" *The Practitioner* 45: 270-279, 322-324.

Pettifor, J.M. 2005. "Rickets" In: Kleerekoper, M, Siris, E. and McChing, M. (eds.) *The Bone and Mineral Manual: A practical guide*. Oxford: Elsevier Academic Press. 39-44.

Railton, T.C. 1894. "Scurvy Rickets" *The Lancet* 143: 532-533.

Ransom, W.B. 1899. "Infant foods and scurvy rickets" *The Lancet* 154: 1256-1257.

Rauch, F. 2003. 'The rachitic bone'. In: Hochberg, Z. (ed.) *Vitamin D and Rickets*. London: Karger. 69-79.

Reginato, A.J. and Coquia, J.A. 2003. Musculoskeletal manifestations of osteomalacia and rickets. *Best Practice and Research Clinical Rheumatology* 17: 1063-1080.

Roberts, C. and Manchester, K. 2005. *The Archaeology of Disease*. New York: Cornell University Press. 221-242.

Seaman, L. and Co. 1869. *Cod-Liver Oil: Its varieties and uses; its purity, mode of preparation, &c*. London: Waterlow and Sons. 5-15.

Smith, R., and Wordsworth, P. 2005. *Clinical and biochemical disorders of the skeleton*. Oxford: Oxford University Press. 173-205.

Smythe, J.R. 1844. *Miscellaneous Contributions to Pathology and Therapeutics; Being a Series of Original Papers on Rickets, Hydrocephalus, Impotence and Sterility, Pulmonary Apoplexy and Haemoptysis.* London: Simplan, Marshall and Co. 1-58.

Snow, S.J. 2006. *Operations without Pain. The Practice and Science of Anaesthesia in Victorian Britain.* Basingstoke: Palgrave Macmillan. 1-9.

Souther, E. 1849. *Facts Interesting to Physicians, Surgeons, Apothecaries, &c. A Treatise on the Use of Cod-liver Oil in the Treatment of Chronic Rheumatism, Scrofula and Consumption, Bronchitis and Asthma, Liver Complaints and all Diseases of the Lungs and Throat* Boston (US): Mead's Press. 1-6.

Stephenson, W. 1865. "Rickets and its pathology clinically considered" *Edinburgh Medical Journal* 10: 611-621.

Wear, A. 1987. "Interfaces: Perceptions of Health and Illness in Early Modern England" In: Porter, R. and Wear, A. (eds.) *Problems and methods in the history of medicine.* Wellcome Institute Series in the History of Medicine. London: Croom Helm. 230-256.

Weinstein, M., Babyn, P. and Zlotkin, S. 2001. "An orange a day keeps the doctor away: Scurvy in the year 2000" *American Academy of Paediatrics* 108: 55-60.

Whyte, M.P. and Thakker, R.V. 2005. "Rickets and osteomalacia". *Medicine* 33: 70-74.

Willmott, W.B. 1860. *Glycerin and Cod-Liver Oil; their History, Introduction, Therapeutic Value and Claims upon Professional and Public Attention.* London: H.Balliére. 91-139.

A morphometric approach to body mass estimation

Lisa Cashmore

Centre for the Archaeology of Human Origins (CAHO), Archaeology,
University of Southampton, Avenue Campus, Southampton, SO17 1BJ
e-mail address for correspondence: lac1@soton.ac.uk

Abstract

Body mass is highly important as it allows a multitude of life history traits to be predicted from a single value. Traditionally, skeletal variables with a biomechanical relationship to body mass have been used to predict weight, but a morphometric approach involving the reconstruction of body size/shape as a cylinder may also prove useful. The aim of this study was to compare the predictive accuracy of bi-iliac diameter as a proxy for the diameter of the cylinder, with another variable that represents body breadth, biacromial diameter. Anthropometric measurements (stature, bi-iliac diameter, biacromial diameter, body mass) were taken from a Papua New Guinean sample of 1017 individuals (477 males and 540 females). The correlation with body mass was assessed using Least Squares regressions based on these measurements. Results showed that, in all analyses, body mass was more strongly correlated with biacromial-based models than when bi-iliac diameter was taken as a measure of body breadth. This suggests that biacromial-based models of body size/shape should be considered where viable for the prediction of body mass, although potential methodological problems need to be addressed.

Keywords: body mass, regression, biacromial, bi-iliac

Introduction

Body mass is one of the most useful variables that can be known about an organism, extant or extinct, as it allows us to predict home range size, relative brain size, sexual dimorphism, taxonomic differences, neonatal weight, and maturation rates (McHenry, 1994) and other life history variables, such as diet, population density and growth, and physiology (Damuth and MacFadden, 1990). Traditionally, body mass has been estimated using standard regression methods such as Least Squares (LS), Reduced Major Axis (RMA), and Major Axis (MA) regression which follow the allometric principle that a change in the size of an independent variable will result in a corresponding and measurable change in the dependant variable (Aiello, 1992; Aiello and Wood, 1994; Smith, 1994). This allows for the prediction of unknown dependant variables such as body mass from known independent variables (for example, bi-iliac diameter). These regression methods often assume a functional relationship between the predictor variable and body mass. Properties of the femur, such as femoral head diameter or midshaft cortical area, are in part constrained by the mechanical role of the femur in transmitting weight through the body. For this reason, it is often assumed that traits that most closely reflect this relationship will be the most reliable predictors of body mass.

Originally designed to investigate the thermoregulatory relationship between body size/shape and climate, Ruff's cylindrical model of the body (Ruff, 1991, 1994) has also been used to predict body mass in both modern humans and hominids (Ruff, 2000; Ruff and Walker, 1993; Ruff et al., 1997; Ruff et al., 2005, Auerbach and Ruff, 2004). Ruff's approach estimates body mass by modelling the body as a cylinder in which stature is the height of the cylinder and bi-iliac diameter is the breadth. This approach removes the functional constraints of weight transmission and focuses on recreating the size and shape of the body. When Ruff and co-workers (Ruff et al., 1997) used this model to predict body mass for Pleistocene *Homo* specimens, they found no statistical difference between body mass as predicted by the model and the values predicted by femoral head breadth (see also Auerbach and Ruff, 2004). Ruff justifies his choice of bi-iliac diameter as a proxy for body breadth on the basis that this variable is commonly present and measurable in large numbers of both skeletal and living samples, has low measurement error, low dependence on limb morphology, and there is a direct comparison between living and fossil samples (assuming similar adaptations to bipedalism). Neither biacromial diameter or bitrochanter diameter have been used in Ruff's research as a breadth measurement and therefore it remains uncertain whether using biacromial diameter would improve the efficacy of body mass predictions.

The aim of this study is to compare the efficacy of body mass predictions based on a cylindrical model using bi-iliac diameter as a measure of body breadth, with a cylindrical model using biacromial diameter as an alternative proxy for body breadth, to assess whether alternative measurements of body breadth should be reasonably considered when constructing cylindrical representations of the body.

Materials and methods

The data used in this study was taken from a dataset collected by R. G. Harvey in the late 1960s from the Karkar Island and Lufa Highland regions of New Guinea (Harvey, 1974). Anthropometric variables reflecting the size and shape characteristics of the human body as a cylinder were recorded on a sample of 477 men and 540 women. Stature was taken as the height of the cylinder, while bi-iliac diameter and biacromial diameter were taken as proxies for cylinder breadth. All males in the sample were between 21 and 65 years of age, and all females between 19 and 65 years of age. Harvey's (1974) analysis of growth patterns in these New Guinean populations indicated that males and females generally did not reach final adult height until 21 years and 19 years of age, respectively, and therefore individuals under these ages were excluded from the sample. Individuals over 65 years were also excluded on the basis of Harvey's observation that body mass typically began to decrease after this age in the populations in question (Harvey, 1974). None of the females included in the sample were known to be pregnant. Stature, bi-iliac diameter and biacromial diameter were recorded using the techniques described by Tanner (1964).

A value for the body as a cylinder was calculated using a standard volumetric equation utilised by Ruff (1991):

$$Volume = \frac{\pi}{4}D^2 L \qquad (1)$$

Where D^2 = body breadth
L = body length

This analysis compared the cylindrical model of body mass based on Ruff's model (equation 1) with a coronal plane area model (a simple 2-D rectangle created by multiplying body height by body breadth) to assess their abilities to accurately predict body mass. For each predictor variable both bi-iliac and biacromial diameter were used as a proxy for body breadth. Values for bi-iliac-based cylindrical body volume (CBV1), biacromial-based cylindrical body volume (CBV2), bi-iliac-based coronal plane area (CPA1) and biacromial-based coronal plane area (CPA2) were calculated for each of the subjects in the reference sample.

Least Squares (LS) regressions carried out on the data set to allow comparison of known body mass with each of the morphometric predictor variables. Much debate has focused on the choice of line-fitting model when assessing the relationship between dependent and independent variables (Aiello, 1992; Hartwig-Scherer and Martin, 1992; Aiello and Wood, 1994; Smith, 1994; Hens *et al.*, 2000). The three line-fitting models are known as Major Axis (MA), Reduced Major Axis (RMA), and Least Squares (LS) regression. These models differ in the assumptions they make about whether or not the dependent (x) and independent (y) variables are measured with error. LS (a Model I technique) assumes that the independent variable is measured *without* error (asymmetrical), whereas MA and RMA (both Model II techniques) assumes *both* the x and y variables are sampled *with* error (symmetrical).

Opinion has generally been divided on which of these methods is most suitable for estimating body mass, with the majority of researchers using either RMA or LS regressions (Aiello, 1992; Hartwig-Scherer and Martin, 1992; Aiello and Wood, 1994; Smith, 1994; Hens *et al.*, 2000). RMA in particular is often chosen as it best reflects the central tendency in a bivariate sample, is unaffected by the correlation coefficient, and allows extrapolation beyond the limits of the sample used to generate the prediction equations (Aiello and Wood, 1994). Although RMA or MA may be the most appropriate methods for assessing biomechanical relationships (Aiello, 1992; Smith, 1994), if the purpose of an analysis is for prediction (e.g. weight or stature), then LS is likely to be the most suitable technique. One of the assumptions of LS is that the independent variable is sampled without error, therefore it is also important that both the x and y variables are normally distributed. It has been suggested that LS should only be used if the sample for which predictions are being made falls within the range of the reference sample that was used to generate the prediction (Aiello, 1992). For these reasons, it was decided that a LS regression would be most suitable for the current data set. In addition, stepwise multiple regressions of body mass on bi-iliac diameter and stature, and of body mass on biacromial diameter and stature were also carried out, to provide a comparison to the multiple regressions used to predict body mass by Ruff and Walker (1993).

Results

When the correlations of known body mass with stature, bi-iliac diameter and biacromial diameter are considered, clear differences are observed (Table 1). Biacromial diameter ($R^2 = 0.66$) is far more strongly correlated with body mass than bi-iliac diameter ($R^2 = 0.37$), with stature showing only a slightly weaker correlation than biacromial diameter ($R^2 = 0.61$).

For both bi-iliac diameter and biacromial diameter, CPA variables provide a stronger correlation with body mass than CBV variables (Table 2). Both biacromial-based models (CBV2 and CPA2) also have stronger relationships with body mass than either of the bi-iliac-based models. The comparison for CBV2 and CPA2 (biacromial-based variables) show higher R^2 values than the regression of body mass upon either stature or biacromial diameter alone (Table 1). By contrast, the comparisons for CBV1 and CPA1 (bi-iliac-based variables) have higher R^2 values than the regression of body mass on bi-iliac diameter but lower than that with stature. Both CPA variables and CBV variables are plotted against body mass with a regression line (LS) fitted to each scatterplot (Figs 1 and 2).

Table 1. Least Squares regression statistics comparing known body mass with predictor variables

Predictor variable	N	R^2	Slope	Intercept	F ratio	p
Biacromial diameter	815	0.66	243.4	-32748	1561.4	<0.0001
Stature	1012	0.61	82.4	-77412	1592.5	<0.0001
Bi-iliac diameter	815	0.37	333.9	-36058	482.5	<0.0001

A number of subjects had missing values for certain measurements, thereby reducing some sample sizes

Table 2. Least Squares regression statistics for cylindrical body volume (mm^3 x 10^7) and coronal plane area (mm^3 x 10^7) model predictor variables

Predictor variable	N	R^2	Slope	Intercept	F ratio	p
CBV1 (stature x bi-iliac)	811	0.52	.0004383	12573	851.86	<0.0001
CBV2 (stature x biacromial)	808	0.72	.0002371	16142	2037.80	<0.0001
CPA1 (stature x bi-iliac)	811	0.58	0.156	-12366	1105.58	<0.0001
CPA2 (stature x biacromial)	808	0.74	0.107	-6290	2211.79	<0.0001

Where CBV1 refers to stature x bi-iliac breadth (equation 1), CBV2 to stature x biacromial diameter (equation 1), CPA1 to stature x bi-iliac diameter and CPA2 to stature x biacromial diameter

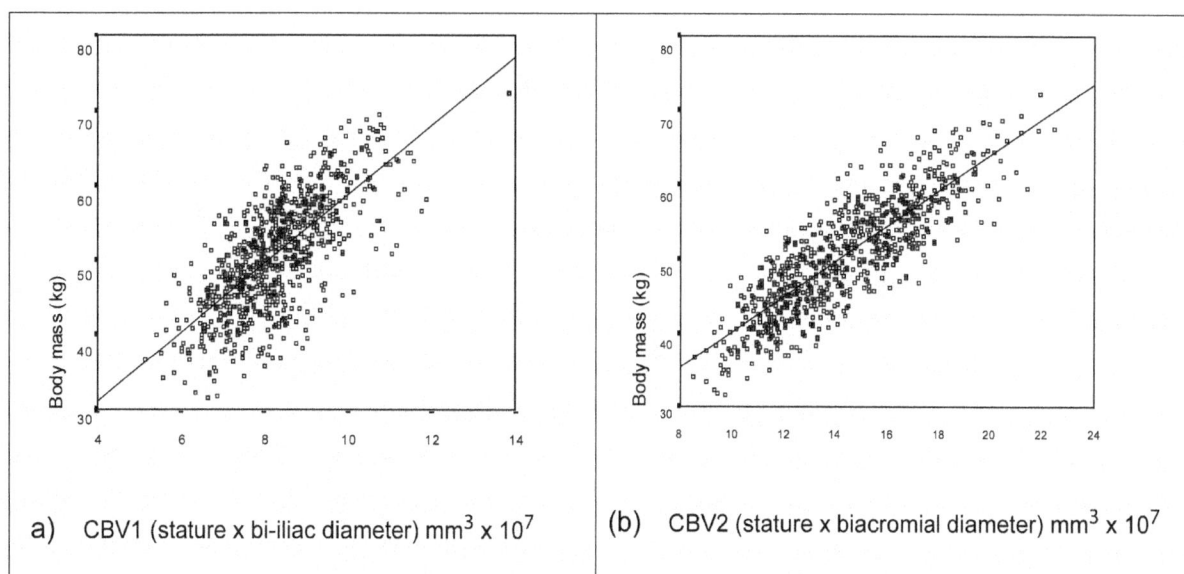

a) CBV1 (stature x bi-iliac diameter) mm^3 x 10^7

(b) CBV2 (stature x biacromial diameter) mm^3 x 10^7

Figure 1. Scatter plots showing the relationships between (a) body mass (kg) and Coronal Plane Area 1 (stature x bi-iliac diameter) (body mass = 0.156 (CPA1) – 12366, R^2=0.58) and (b) body mass (kg) and Coronal Plane Area 2 (stature x biacromial diameter) (body mass = 0.107 (CPA2) – 6290, R^2=0.74). Regression lines (LS) have been added.

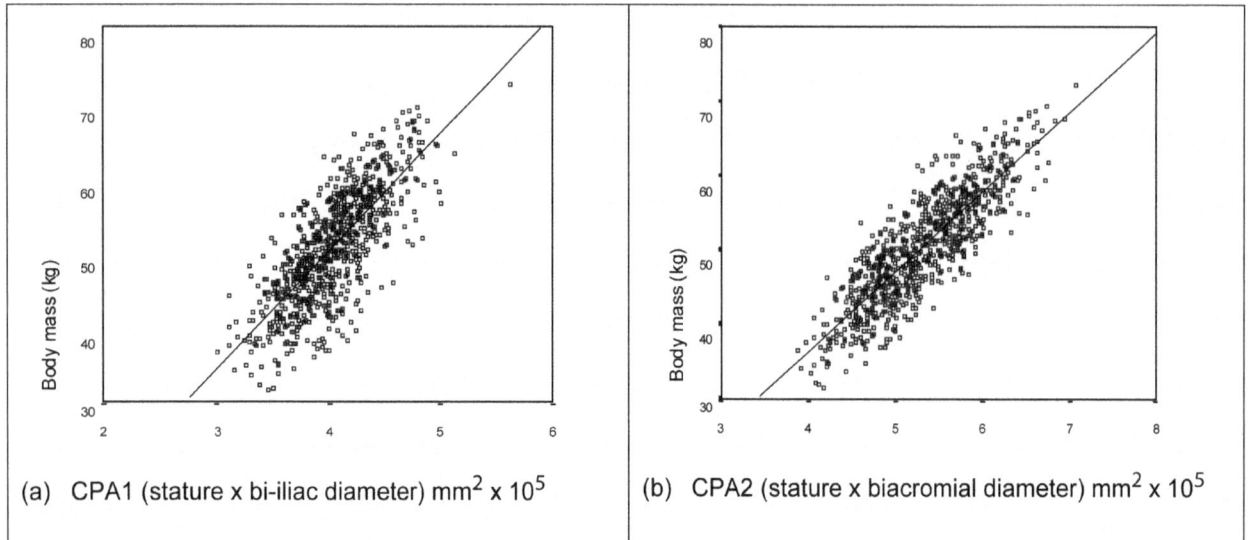

Figure 2. Scatter plots showing the relationships between (a) body mass (kg) and Cylindrical Body Volume 1 (stature x bi-iliac diameter) (body mass = .0004383 (CBV1) + 12573, R^2=0.52) and (b) body mass and Cylindrical Body Volume 2 (stature x biacromial diameter) (body mass = .0002371 (CBV2) + 16142, R^2=0.72). Regression lines (LS) have been added.

When stepwise multiple regressions were carried out on stature and bi-iliac and biacromial diameters, the results were found to be very similar to those of the standard LS regression (Table 3). For the biacromial-based regressions in particular, there was little difference between the techniques and therefore no one method can be recommended over the other. For the bi-iliac-based regressions however, the difference was greater. This suggests that if bi-iliac diameter is used as a measure of breadth, then a multiple regression may provide more reliable estimations of body mass than a standard linear regression based on a cylinder- or coronal plane area-based model.

Table 3. Least Squares regression statistics for stepwise multiple regressions of stature (mm) and bi-iliac diameter (mm), and stature (mm) and biacromial diameter (mm).

Regression variables	N	R^2	Slope	Intercept
Stature + bi-iliac diameter	811	0.62	stature = 68.5 bi-iliac = 99.2	-81440
Stature + biacromial diameter	808	0.72	stature = 151.77 biacromial = 41.61	-65901

Discussion

The results of this analysis suggest that further attention should be paid to the use of cylindrical models of the body, such as that adopted by Ruff (1991, 1994, 2000; Ruff and Walker, 1993; Ruff et al., 1997; Ruff et al., 2005; Auerbach and Ruff, 2004) in predicting body mass for hominids. Ruff's model uses stature to represent the height of the cylinder and bi-iliac diameter to represent breadth. There is potential, however, for alternative

skeletal measurements, such as biacromial diameter, to accurately represent cylinder breadth. In this analysis, biacromial diameter-based models of body size were more strongly correlated with body mass than bi-iliac diameter-based models (Table 2). Both CPA models performed better in this respect than either of the CBV models, although the reason for this is unclear at present. Multiple regressions of body mass on bi-iliac diameter and stature and of biacromial diameter and stature had higher R^2 values than simple regressions of body mass upon stature and either bi-iliac diameter or biacromial diameter respectively (Table 3). The stature and bi-iliac diameter regression had a stronger correlation than both CBV1 and CPA1. The stature and biacromial diameter regression performed as well as CBV2, but not better than CPA2 (although the difference was slight). Both Jungers (1990) and Smith (1996) have advocated the use of multiple regression and the current results suggest that, where possible, this approach should be explored.

This current study suggests bi-iliac diameter may not be the most statistically reliable proxy for body breadth and that, in this sample, biacromial diameter can be considered as an alternative when generating cylindrical models of body size/shape. Therefore, where possible, biacromial diameter should be included, along with bi-iliac diameter, in the construction of the cylindrical model. Despite Smith's (2002) assurance that the statistical quality of a predictor variable is more important than factors such as functional relationships, the use of biacromial diameter as a proxy for body breadth should be approached with caution. When measured in living samples biacromial diameter is likely to exhibit more interobserver measurement error than bi-iliac diameter (Bennett and Osborne, 1986) and this error is likely to increase when this measurement is taken on skeletal samples, due to the difficulty of accurately reconstructing the pectoral girdle. However, a reasonable correlation between the bi-iliac based models and body mass was still found, which should be considered along with the comparative ease of reconstructing the pelvis in skeletal samples. When these factors are taken together it suggests that, while biacromial diameter may provide a more accurate representation of the breadth of the human body, methodological issues may preclude its use as a component of the cylindrical model. If this is the case then it may be more appropriate to use bi-iliac diameter as a proxy for body breadth, as suggested by Ruff (Ruff and Walker, 1993).

While Ruff used a geographically diverse sample to construct his cylindrical model, the current study uses a sample that is derived solely from a Papua New Guinea population (Harvey, 1974). This reduced geographical variability needs to be taken into consideration when applying the results of this study to other populations if it is shown that subjects exhibit different body plans from the Papua New Guinea sample. It may be that the relationship between biacromial diameter, stature and body mass varies across geographical areas and therefore a possible avenue of future research would be to incorporate data from more geographically dispersed subjects in order to test the performance of biacromial diameter as a proxy for body breadth when compared to bi-iliac diameter.

Conclusion

Biacromial diameter, an alternative measurement of body breadth, was found to be more strongly correlated with body mass than the more widely used proxy bi-iliac diameter. When biacromial diameter was used to represent body breadth in a cylindrical model of body size/shape (as used by Ruff, 1991 and subsequent papers), this breadth measurement was once again found to be more strongly correlated with body mass than cylindrical models based on bi-iliac diameter. An alternative model of body size/shape, based on a simple 2-D representation of the body as a rectangle, showed a better correlation with body mass than Ruff's more commonly used volumetric model. Stepwise multiple regressions of stature and bi-iliac diameter and stature and biacromial diameter on body mass performed better than either of the morphometric models. While these results suggest that biacromial diameter is a more suitable proxy for body breadth than bi-iliac diameter, caution should be exercised when using this measurement to construct a cylindrical model, due to problems in accurately measuring this trait in skeletal samples.

Literature cited

Aiello, L.C. 1992. "Allometry and the analysis of size and shape in human evolution" *Journal of Human Evolution* 22: 127–147.

Aiello, L.C. and Wood, B.A. 1994. "Cranial variables as predictors of hominine body mass" *American Journal of Physical Anthropology* 93: 409–426.

Auerbach, B.M. and Ruff, C.B. 2004. "Human body mass estimation: A comparison of "morphometric" and "mechanical" methods" *American Journal of Physical Anthropology* 125: 331–342.

Bennett, K.A. and Osborne, R.H. 1986. "Interobserver measurement reliability in anthropology" *Human Biology* 5: 751-759.

Damuth, J. and MacFadden, B.J. 1990. "Introduction: body size and its estimation". In: Damuth, J. and MacFadden, B.J. (eds.) *Body Size in Mammalian Paleobiology: Estimation and Biological Implications.* Cambridge: Cambridge University Press. 1–8.

Hartwig-Scherer, S. and Martin, R.D. 1992. "Allometry and prediction in hominoids: A solution to the problem of intervening variables" *American Journal of Physical Anthropology* 88: 37–57.

Harvey, R.G. 1974. "An anthropometric survey of growth and physique of the populations of Karkar Island and Lufa subdistrict, New Guinea" *Philosophical Transactions of the Royal Society of London: B* 268: 279–292.

Hens, S.M., Konigsberg, L.W. and Jungers, W.L. 2000. "Estimating stature in fossil hominids: which regression model and reference sample to use?" *Journal of Human Evolution* 38: 767–784.

Jungers, W.L. 1990. "Problems and methods in reconstructing body size in fossil primates". In: Damuth, J. and MacFadden, B.J. (eds.) *Body Size in Mammalian Paleobiology: Estimation and Biological Implications.* Cambridge: Cambridge University Press. 103–117.

McHenry, H.M. 1994. "Behavioral ecological implications of early hominid body size" *Journal of Human Evolution* 27: 77–87.

Ruff, C.B. 1991. "Climate and body shape in hominid evolution" *Journal of Human Evolution* 21: 81–105.

Ruff, C.B. 1994. "Morphological adaptation to climate in modern and fossil hominids" *Yearbook of Physical Anthropology* 37: 65–107.

Ruff, C.B. 2000. "Body mass prediction from skeletal frame size in elite athletes" *American Journal of Physical Anthropology* 113: 507–517.

Ruff, C.B., Niskanen, M., Junno, J.A. and Jamison, P. 2005. "Body mass prediction from stature and bi-iliac breadth in two high latitude populations, with application to earlier higher latitude humans" *Journal of Human Evolution* 48: 381–392.

Ruff, C.B., Trinkaus, E. and Holliday, T.W. 1997. "Body mass and encephalization in Pleistocene *Homo*" *Nature* 387: 173–176.

Ruff, C.B. and Walker, A. 1993. "Body size and body shape". In: Walker, A. and Leakey, R. (eds.) *The Nariokotome Homo erectus skeleton.* Berlin: Springer – Verlag. 234–265.

Smith, R.J. 1994. "Current events: Regression models for prediction equations" *Journal of Human Evolution* 26: 239–244.

Smith, R.J. 1996. "Biology and body size in human evolution: Statistical inference misapplied" *Current Anthropology* 37: 451–481.

Smith, R.J. 2002. "Estimation of body mass in paleontology" *Journal of Human Evolution* 42: 271–287.

Tanner, J.M. 1964. *The Physique of the Olympic Athlete.* London: George Allen and Unwin Ltd.

Lacunae to fill: combining palaeopathological and documentary research in investigations of individuals from a post-medieval Swedish cemetery

Caroline Arcini

National Heritage Board, UV SYD, 226 60 Lund, Sweden
e-mail address for correspondence: caroline.arcini@raa.se

Abstract

When a part of the cemetery belonging to the cathedral of Linköping in Sweden was excavated in 2002 and 2003 an opportunity arose to compare written sources to data derived from osteoarchaeological sources. The cemetery was in use from 1100 to 1810 and changes in burial customs during these 700 years made it possible to divide the material into three burial periods. A number of written sources were available including the Swedish national registration system. The national registration system contained a wealth of information on an individual basis, such as cause of death, age at death, number of children, matrimonial age, social status etc. The principal focus of the material presented in this paper is the last burial period (1780-1810) and specifically the problems and results related to the identification of individuals from the site, providing a fuller picture of a past community.

Keywords: Cathedral of Linköping, cemetery, human osteology, historical sources, tuberculosis, syphilis.

Introduction

For periods prior to the introduction of official registration of births, marriages and deaths in 1686, archaeological human remains provide the main source of information on health and disease in Sweden, both at an individual and an aggregate level. When studying the living conditions and patterns of health in ancient societies this information is of great importance. In Sweden over the last couple of decades archaeological skeletal material from historic periods has become accessible, and occasionally written records that can be linked to the skeletal remains are available. Can comparisons of results from these two sources make a significant contribution to knowledge of the actual period, and also be used as a tool to interpret results from periods where no written sources are available? The written records, can for example, reveal relatively exact information about age at death distribution and what diseases we can expect to find in the bones and teeth. This paper serves to illustrate some of the problems of attempting to combine written and paleopathological evidence. The two main questions are: 1) Is it possible to trace and identify individuals, comparing certain diseases or disabilities manifested in the skeletal material with information from written records; 2) Is it possible to calculate how many cases of a condition we could expect to find in skeletal materials from the known frequency of diseases in the register such as tuberculosis. A more detailed presentation of the paleopathological findings from this collection will follow in a later publication.

Materials and methods

In 2002-3 excavations were carried out of a part of the cemetery belonging to the Cathedral of Linköping, Sweden (Figs. 1 and 2). The cemetery was in use from ca.1100 to1810 A.D. and changes in burial customs over this time allow the 570 burials excavated to be divided into three broad periods. In this paper only the graves excavated from the latest burial period, 1780-1810 A.D., will be discussed. This cemetery is unique in Sweden, as in addition to data derived from analysis of the human remains there are also several contemporary written sources, such as church registers, catechetical meeting records and letters from the medical doctor in the town.

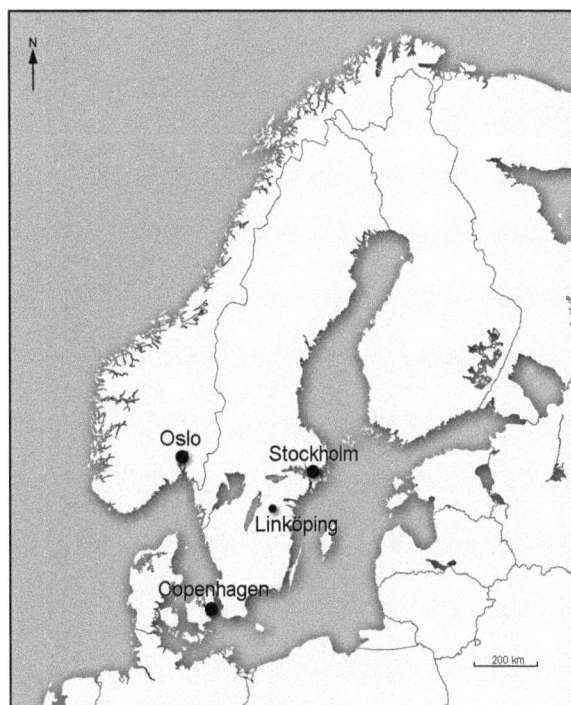

Figure1. Map of Sweden showing location of Linköping, south west of Stockholm.

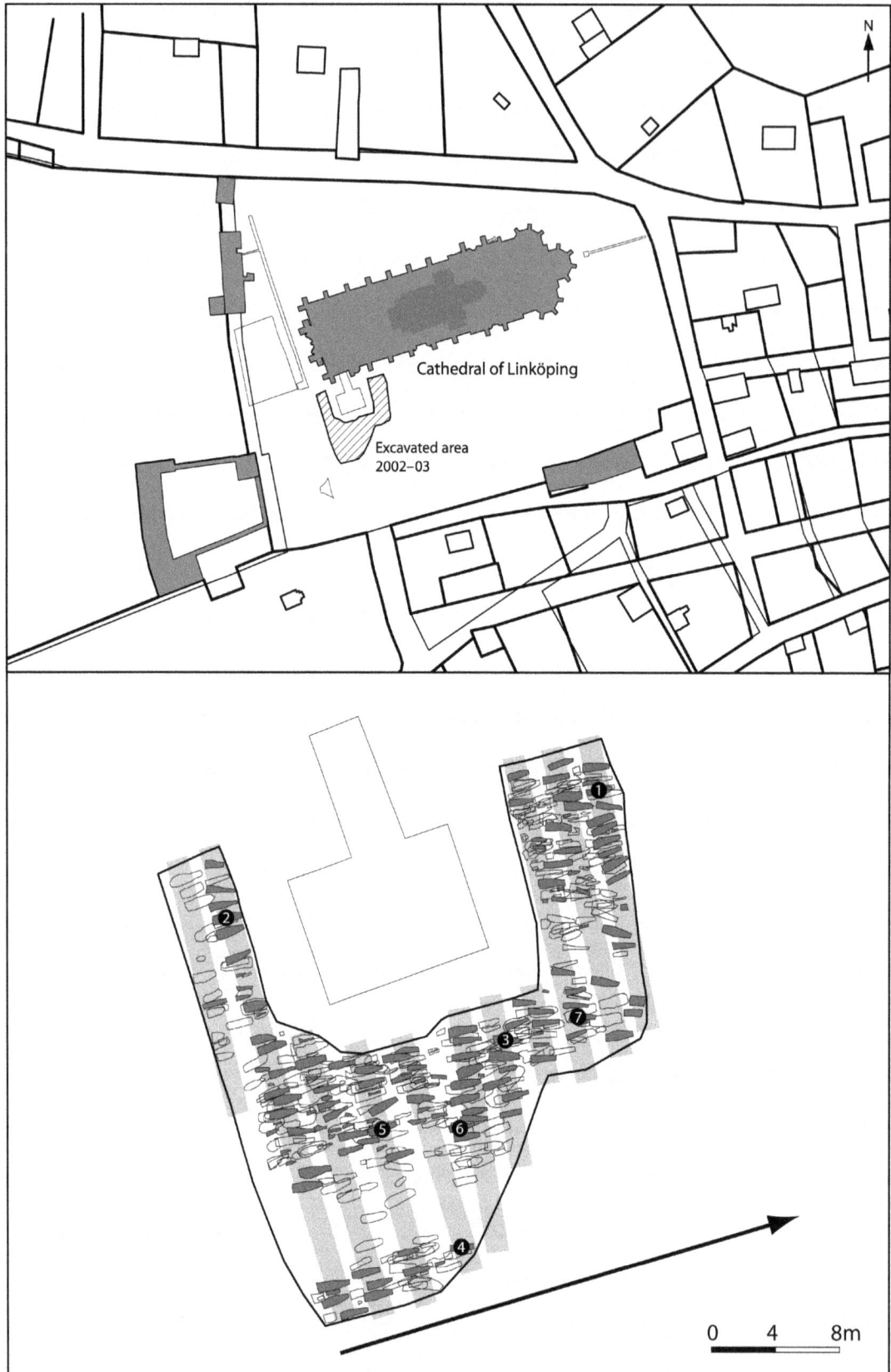

Figure 2. Plan of the Cathedral of Linköping with cemetery. The hatched area shows the excavated part of the cemetery. The lower image shows a plan of the burial lines. According to the new policy, all individuals should be buried on a line and gravediggers started the lines in the western part of the cemetery, progressing towards the eastern wall (in the direction of the arrow). #1: Woman buried together with a newborn baby. #2: Woman with suspected cystic tuberculosis. #3: Woman with severe syphilitic changes, possibly the individual that died in 1786. #4: Woman with syphilitic changes, possibly the individual that died in 1795. #5: Coin made 1802 to 1808 found in the grave. #6: Coin made after 1800 found in the grave. #7: Earrings made after 1801 found on the skeleton.

Swedish church registers include information such as cause of death, age at death and information about the time between death and burial. There is also information about circumstances that negated burial in the ordinary cemetery and what the alternatives were. For example, individuals may have been buried at the place of execution, the woods, or in the northern part of the cemetery. The church register also contains a number of important details regarding burial customs. There are for instance examples of two individuals being buried in the same grave or even in the same coffin. The civil status and information on family relations of the individual are also noted.

Another source that can give valuable information is the notes made by the priest during the parish catechetical meetings, i.e. yearly meetings held in the homes of the parishioners where the priest interrogates them on their knowledge of Christianity. These notes could also contain information about an individual's diseases or disabilities. Things that might be noted included if the person had one leg shorter than the other, were deaf, had a physical or psychological disability or if they had an incurable or venereal disease. More than 35,000 notes have been analysed from such meetings held in Linköping during the time period relating to the excavated burials.

The third documentary source that the project has access to is the letters from the district medical officer Johan Otto Hagström. During his time as a doctor (1747-1791) he wrote approximately 300 letters both to *Collegium Medicum* in Stockholm, and Abraham Bäck (Hagström, 1993, 1997). The letters contain among many other things, information about the health situation, medical treatment, epidemics, local weather, harvest situation, local food prices in Linköping and the county of Östergötland.

Ageing and sexing were carried out according to standards proposed by Buikstra and Ubelaker (1994). After analysing the skeletal material, the Department of History at the University of Linköping and the University of Umeå provided access to their huge demographic databases. These databases contain church registers and the notes from the catechetical meetings in digital form.

Results

Of the 570 excavated graves from this cemetery, about 140 dated between 1780-1810. The bone preservation of the skeletons from this period was not as good at that from the earlier periods and some skeletal areas had been destroyed by adipocere. According to the church registers the cemetery was initially divided into various sections for different groups or families. For example, the people working at the school had their burial place close to the bell tower. The poor also had their special section, the western part of the cemetery, which was also the place that was first used when the plague struck Linköping in 1710.

However, in 1780 in Linköping, as in many other cities of Sweden, family plots were abolished and it also became more difficult for the wealthy to buy new graves inside the church. Exceptions were made for those who already had family graves in the church, which they could continue to use. This new policy stated that all individuals should be buried in lines independent of age, sex, social status or family relations (Hassler, 1976). These changes were introduced because it had become very crowded in some parts of the cemetery and below the church floor.

When the excavation started the archaeologist quickly noticed that several of the graves formed lines, (Fig. 2). Some of the lines were straighter than others and some graves are placed very close to each other. From the written sources it is known that the gravediggers began burying along the west part of the cemetery and when they reached the eastern end of the cemetery wall, they started all over again (Fig. 2) (Hassler, 1976). With few exceptions the individuals were buried in wooden coffins, and in some cases, the iron handles of the coffins of the wealthier persons survived. Buttons and fragments of different materials showed that several were buried dressed in clothes made of silk, fine woven wool, leather gloves and some were wearing their personal belongings such as earrings and finger rings. Traces of bridal wreaths made from copper thread and cowberry leaves revealed that girls, even the newborn and unmarried women, were dressed as the bride they had never had the opportunity to become (Fig. 3). The custom with the bridal wreath spread from Germany to Denmark and by the 17th century it had reached Sweden (Hagberg, 1937).

The cemetery was used by two parishes; one belonging to the Cathedral and the other to the church of St Lars. According to the National Registration Records they had around 4000 parishioners during this time period. About 150-170 of them died each year. This means that during the period 1780-1810 about 4500 individuals were buried, in lines, in this cemetery. Figure 4 presents a comparison of data on the known average age distribution of these individuals from written sources and that derived from the osteological analysis of the skeletal material. It shows that the proportion of subadults is more or less the same in the two sources. The main difference is shown among adult individuals. According to the written sources only 14% died between 20 – 39 years of age, but the osteological data indicates that this figure was 35%. In the oldest adults, those over 60 years of age, the pattern seen is almost the reverse with far more older adults recorded in the church register than the skeletal material.

Efforts made to identify some of the individuals are ongoing, but so far efforts have been concentrated on three different phenomena. The first is complications in childbirth, where we ought expect to find a woman of fertile age buried together with an infant in the same coffin. The second is phthisis (i.e. tuberculosis) shown by traces of chronic bacterial infection in the bones, especially in the spine. The third is venereal disease such

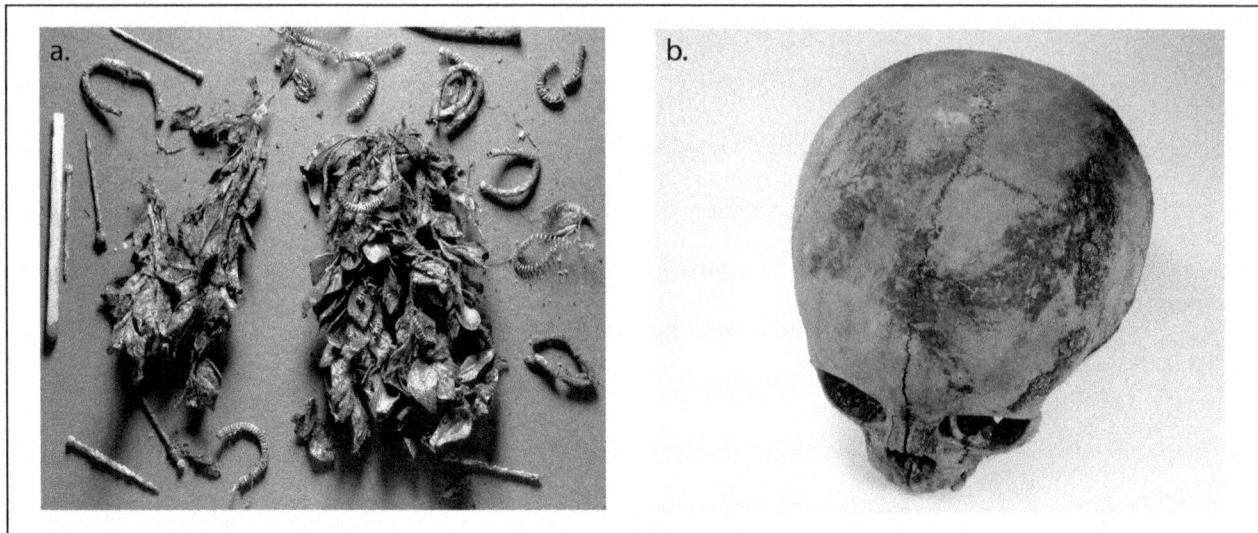

Figure 3. a.) Parts of bridal wreaths made from copper thread and cowberry leaves; b.) Sub-adult skull, the darker areas visible are in reality green, having been stained by copper thread from a bridal wreath.

as syphilis, which manifests in the skeleton during the tertiary stage of the disease.

In the archaeological material one grave contained an adult woman who was assumed to be married, as there was no evidence of a wreath. She was about 20 - 25 years of age and was buried in the same coffin as a newborn infant (Fig. 2, #1). The infant was placed in her arms. Analysis of the documentary sources has identified eight cases where a mother and her newborn baby were buried on the same day. In four of these cases, it was specifically mentioned that they were buried in the same coffin. In only two of the cases identified, was the mother younger than 35 years of age. Since we know the age and sex of those who died and were buried before and after the woman and her child on the line, it should be possible to find out which of the archaeological cases it represents. However, several individuals were buried on the same day and in those cases it was necessary to compare a lot of different combinations from the church registers (Table 1).

Identifying specific individuals with tuberculosis proved to be far more difficult. The church register revealed that tuberculosis was a common disease, so there were more probable cases to look through. From the approximate number of cases of tuberculosis found in the written material so far, it is possible to calculate the number that could be expected in the skeletal material analysed. Before the introduction of antibiotics, the frequency of skeletal tuberculosis was about 5-7% of those who were affected by the condition, and about 1-3.5 % of these could be expected to have had changes in the spine (Steinbock, 1976; Zimmerman and Kelly, 1982; Strouhal, 1988). Of the 4529 individuals that died between 1780-1810, there were 362 individuals (8%); where tuberculosis were the probable cause of death. This means that if we had access to all the 4529 skeletons we could expect between 18 and 25 individuals to display skeletal manifestations and between seven and 11

individuals to have changes in the spine.

The excavated skeletal material comprised of 140 individuals, which means that it would be reasonable to expect one case. Only one case with changes in the spine indicative of tuberculosis, i.e. Pott's disease (Fig. 5) was found in the skeletal material. It is of a young married woman who died when she was about 20 - 25 years of age (Fig. 2, #2). However, the skeleton also shows other changes resulting from a chronic form of osteomyelitis (Fig. 6). Spondylitic changes were present at three places in the spine; the atlas, thoracic vertebrae 5, 6 and 12, and the first and second lumbar vertebrae. The destruction of the twelfth thoracic and first and second lumbar vertebrae resulted in a typical Pott's hump. There were also bilateral osteomyelitic changes on the clavicles and scapulae, with sequestration of the right clavicle. Changes on the ribs, left ulna, both femora and tibiae and fibulae also appeared typical of those described by Resnick and Niawayama (1989) relating to a rare form of tuberculosis

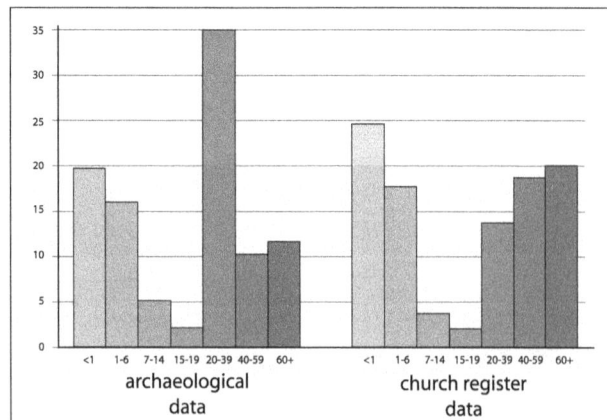

Figure 4. The age distribution from the osteological analysis of the skeletal material compared to the known average age distribution of these individuals based on historical records.

Table 1. Sample of information obtained from church registers used in attempts to identify excavated individuals.

Name	Date of death	Date of burial	Age			Cause of death	Funeral circumstances
			Years	Months	Days		
Nils	1795 08 01	1795 08 09	0	0	5	Slag*	
Anna Catharina Lindahl	1795 08 11	1795 08 16	35	0	0	Childbirth	
Peter	1795 08 12	1795 08 16	0	0	17	Slag*	Buried with mother in same coffin
Eva Maria	1795 08 13	1795 08 18	9	0	0	TB	
Christina Lovisa	1795 08 24	1795 08 27	3	0	24	Smallpox	

*Swedish medical term referring to 'convulsions causing unconsciousness'.

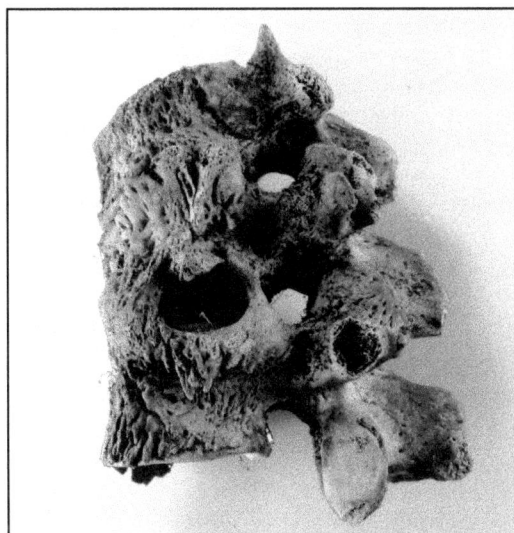

Figure 5. Changes due to tuberculosis (Pott's disease).

According to Resnick and Niawayama (1989) there is a form of tuberculosis called cystic tuberculosis osteomyelitis, a rare variety more frequent in children than in adults. Cystic tuberculosis osteomyelitis might be a possible diagnosis for the changes recorded in this young woman. This condition is associated with cystic lesions, and the radiographic characteristics include well-defined osseous lesions that resemble those of eosinophilic granuloma, sarcoidosis, cystic angiomatosis, plasma cell myeloma, fungal infection, metastases and other conditions. Severe enamel hypoplasias on numerous teeth reveal that the young woman might have had a several intermittent recurrences of the disease in early childhood. However, much more research is needed before it is possible to suggest a probable identity to this woman.

The third attempt to identify individuals concerns two female individuals with syphilis. One is a married woman, who is estimated to have been between 30 - 40 years of age when she died (Fig. 2, #3). In addition to the changes on the bones of the arms and legs, she also had severe syphilitic changes on the frontal bone (i.e. caries sicca) and on the left maxilla (Figs. 7 and 8). These bone lesions suggest extensive skin wounds including a large

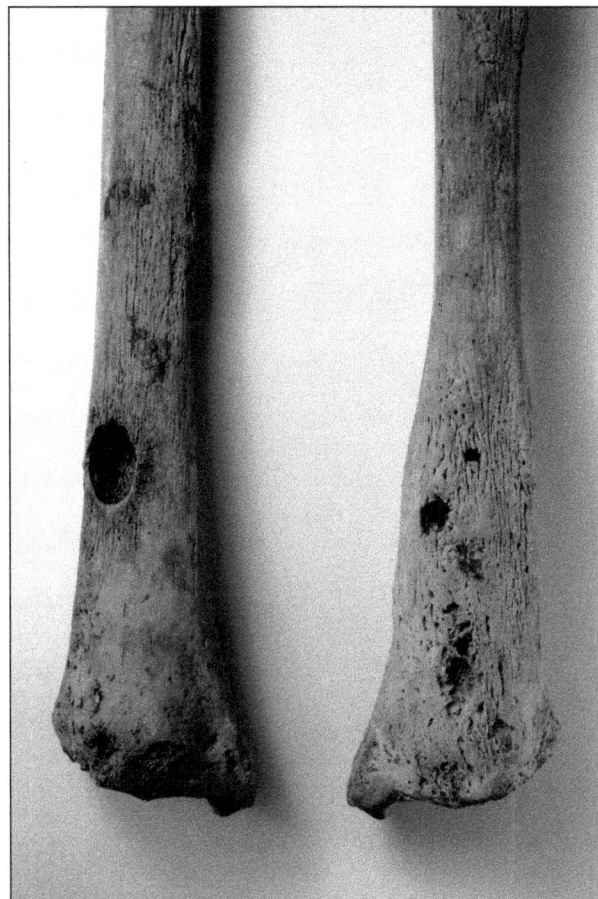

Figure 6. Changes due to cystic tuberculosis osteomyelitis on the tibiae.

part of her forehead, which would have been impossible to hide. The other woman, who was unmarried, was estimated to have died at the age of 25 - 30 years (Fig. 2, #4). In her case it seems that the disease was not as severe on the skull, but there were extensive lesions on the bones of the leg. Since the changes that can be observed in the skeletons show the tertiary stage of the disease, the individuals and the community must have been aware of their disease for several years.

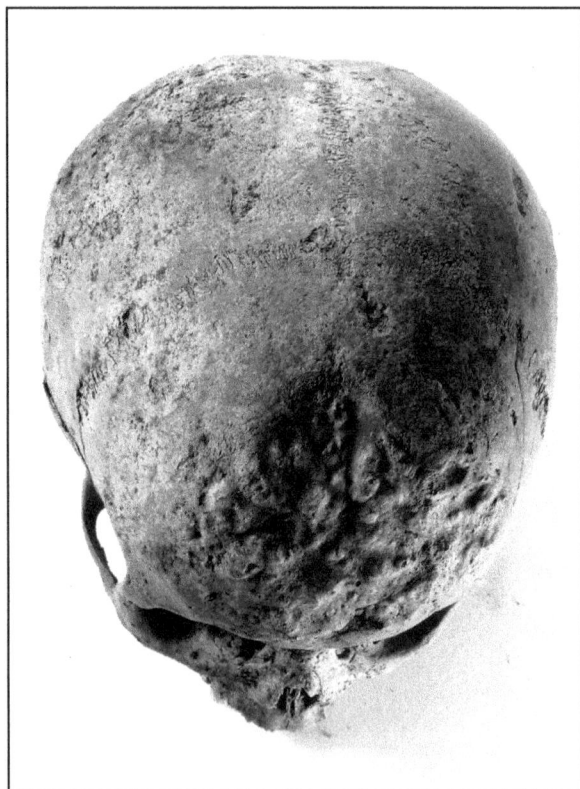

Figure 7. Typical syphilitic changes on the frontal bone.

Examination of the church registers for the period 1780-1810 A.D. revealed that there were two women, two men and a sub-adult girl whose cause of death was diagnosed as venereal disease. According to the church register one of the women was unmarried and 27 years when she died and the other was 35 and married. Could these perhaps be the two women from the archaeological material? One problem is that according to the church register the younger one died in 1795 and the older woman in 1786, but the earlier burial is to the west of the later one (Fig. 2). Examination of other skeletons in the line where these two women were buried did not help, as the lines were not particularly straight. There were also circumstances during the archaeological excavation, which resulted in the loss of skeletons in the area around the younger woman. In an attempt to understand the lines, the datable finds from the excavation was analysed. There were coins that were made after 1800 (Fig. 2 #5 and #6) and one pair of earrings (Fig. 2 #7) that we know from the initials had been made by the silversmith Henrik Hervander, who worked in Linköping during 1801-1823 (Arcini and Tagesson, 2005).

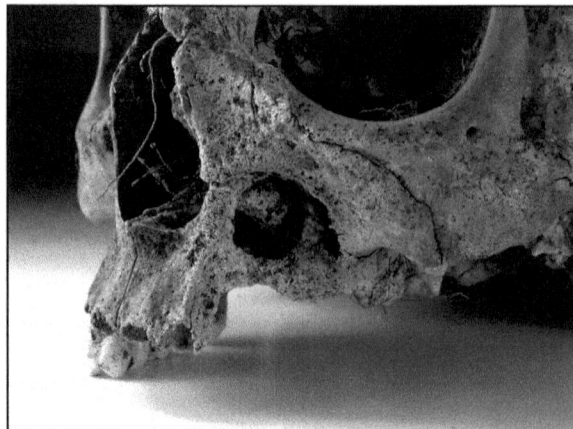

Figure 8. Traces of a syphilitic lesion on the left maxilla.

The results showed that the two coins and the pair of earrings manufactured after 1800 were found in graves from lines both west and east of the individuals affected by syphilis (Fig. 2 #3 and #4). One explanation for this could be that the line system was not abruptly introduced over the cemetery or strictly adhered to. At the introduction of the new burial mode, gravediggers had to pay respect to recent graves. Therefore, they had to first fill the spaces between family and earlier groups of graves. When they reached the eastern part of the cemetery wall some ten or 20 years later, they started all over again. That is why we find coins in graves from earlier western lines minted after 1800.

Discussion

The focus of this paper has been to present the initial results of efforts to combine osteoarchaeological material with the available written sources from a cemetery in Sweden. The first aspect presented was the differences found between osteological results and the written sources regarding the age distribution for the adults. Ever since the investigation of the Christ Church Spitalfields material from London showed that as much as 42% of the adults were estimated to be younger than they were (Molleson *et al.*, 1993), we have been aware of that there really are problems with the age estimation of older adult individuals. Even though the current data does not provide information on the age of each individual like in the Spitalfields material, information on the age distribution of adult individuals follows the same broad pattern as that found in the investigation at Spitalfields. Of course it could be argued that the individuals analysed as part of the current investigations do not represent an average of the 4,529 people that died and were recorded in the documentary sources. However, there are no indications that juveniles were over-represented. For the development of osteology it is crucial that further research into this issue is carried out, perhaps inspired by work in recent material with known age especially of old people, to find better methods.

It is clear that further research is required on the identification of specific individuals. This is very time consuming work as there are many possibilities, and the

Demographic Database from Umeå University is not searchable in that way. However, the two cases of syphilis might very well be those found in the church register. In addition, what are the chances that these two women severely affected by syphilis, were able to live unnoticed in a town like Linköping? Many of the letters from the district medical doctor, Hagström, make it clear that venereal syphilis was a serious problem for the people of his district (Hagström, 1993, 1997). It was not only the disease that was painful, the shame and the stigma was also a huge problem. If people were suspected of suffering from the disease, they were not allowed to visit the church and sometimes the whole family had to leave their home and the village, even though only one person in the family was affected (Hagström, 1993 and 1997). Some even changed their names before they moved into another village. Even those who recovered had problems and Hagström mentioned two cases where the individuals committed suicide, they could not bear the shame.

Hagström also mentions that sometimes when he met people in the market they did not want him to recognise them, because others could interpret it as meaning that he had treated them for venereal disease. It is also mentioned in several of his letters that it is impossible to get a room in the city for a person while he treats them. According to the very simple medical records compiled by the hospital, most beds were occupied by people with venereal disease (1998). However, several recovered and died of other causes (Hagström, 1993, 1997). That as much as 65% of those affected by syphilis in the first and second stage really could recover without medical treatment were confirmed in the Oslo study (Gjestland, 1955).

So, was it possible during these circumstances, for these two women to escape notice by the priest? It is very likely that the 30 - 40 year old woman died from complications due to syphilis and therefore, the cause of death would have been venereal disease. As today it was the doctor who stated the cause of death and in those days the priest had the obligation to report it to the Collegium Medicum. Of course since it was such a shame to have had the disease a wealthy individual could have tried to hide it and asked the doctor to give another cause of death. However, in this case they would have had to hide the woman for several years. As the age, sex and social status fits, it is likely that the two women with syphilitic changes are the first identified individuals from this cemetery.

The identification of pathological individuals will be of tremendous help in understanding how different diseases manifest themselves and the degree of variation in their appearance. We may also find traces on the skeletons that we do not recognise because people today have treatment before it affects the bones. It will enable us to identify the circumstances concerning age determination of old adult individuals. As we reuse more areas in the modern cities, late historical cemeteries will be subjected to exploitation and it is important to stress the significance these types of material can have in interpreting life conditions in earlier societies.

This paper has shown that there are several "lacunae to fill". When the gravediggers had to follow the new burial custom, to bury the dead in lines, they had to fill the spaces between the earlier graves. The osteologist, archaeologists and historians have also found that with co-operation they can link together the results from their different sources and fill several spaces. Finally, the new knowledge that would be gained about life conditions in Linköping 200 years ago will hopefully be applicable in the interpretation of circumstances 400 or 900 years ago.

Acknowledgments

The author is grateful to Staffan Hyll, National Heritage Board UV SYD, for photographs and graphics, and to Göran Tagesson, National Heritage Board UV Öst, the archaeologist in charge of the excavation, for discussions about the burial customs. The National Heritage Board UV SYD provided funds for the BABAO conference in Birmingham. Annica Cardell, National Heritage Board UV Syd, and Torbjörn Ahlström, University of Lund, for discussions and revisions of the text. Sören Edvinsson and Anna Lundberg at The Demographical Database, University of Umeå, for access to the demographic database of Linköping. Ingrid Olsson, Marie C. Nelson and Hans Nilsson, University of Linköping, for historical data concerning the town of Linköping and its inhabitants. Funding from the Research and Development programme of the National Heritage Board made it possible to utilise the historical sources. Thanks also to Megan Brickley, University of Birmingham for improving the manuscript.

Literature cited

Arcini, C. and Tagesson, G. 2005. "Kroppen som materiell kultur. Gravar och människor genom 700 år". In: Liunga. Kaupinga. *Kulturhistoria och arkeologi i Linköpin.*

Buikstra, J.E. and Ubelaker, D.H., (eds.) 1994. *Standards for Data Collection from Human Skeletal Remains.* Arkansas: Arkansas Archaeological Survey Research Series No. 44.

Gjestland, T. 1955. "The Oslo study of untreated syphilis, an epidemiological gsbygden". In: Kaliff, A. and Tagesson, G. (eds.) "Investigation of the natural course of the syphilitic infection based upon a re-study of the Boeck-Brusgaard Material" *Acta Dermato-Venereologica* 35, supp. 34: 3-368.

Hagberg, L. 1937. *När döden gästar. Svenska folkseder och svensk folktro i samband med död och begravning.* Stockholm: Wahlström and Widstrand.

Hagström, J.O. 1993. *Johan Otto Hagströms brev till Collegium Medicum 1755-1785.* Östergötlands: Medicinhistoriska Sällskap.

Hagström, J.O. 1997 *"Välborne Herr Archiater..."* Johan Otto Hagströms brev till Abraham Bäck 1747-1791. Östergötlands: Medicinhistoriska Sällskap.

Hassler, O. 1976. *Kyrkogården berättar om det Linköping som var.* Linköpings och S:t Lars griftegård 1811-1899.

Lundberg, A. 1998. " 'Läkta till samhällets tjänst' - veneriska sjukdomar, läkare och botande i Östergötland 1770-1838" *Svensk Medicinhistorisk Tidskrift* 2: 29-48.

Molleson, T., Cox, M., Waldron, A.H. and Whittaker, D.K. 1993. *The Spitalfields Project: the Middling Sort. Vol 2 – the Anthropology.* York: Council for British Archaeology.

Resnick, D. and Niawayama, G. 1989. *Diagnosis of Bone and Joint Disorders.* Philadelphia: W.B. Saunders.

Steinbock, T.R. 1976. *Paleopathological diagnosis and interpretation: bone diseases in ancient human populations.* Springfield, Illinois: Charles C. Thomas.

Strouhal, E. 1988. "Vertebral tuberculosis in ancient Egypt and Nubia". In: Ortner, D.J. and Aufterheide, A.C. (eds.) *Human Paleopathology Current Synthesis and Future Option.* Washington: Smithsonian Institution Press.

Zimmerman, M.R. and Kelly, M.A. 1982. *Atlas of Human Paleopathology.* New York: Praeger.

Tuberculosis of the shoulder in a Victorian girl: how the invention of radiographs overturned a diagnosis of hysteria

Amna Suliman[1] and Piers D. Mitchell[2]*

[1]Undergraduate Medical Office, Imperial College London, Reynolds Building, Room 138,
St Dunstan's Road, London, W6 8RP
[2]Imperial College London, 7 East, Charing Cross Hospital,
Fulham Palace Road, London, W6 8RF
*e-mail address for correspondence: piers.mitchell@imperial.ac.uk

Abstract

In 19th century Britain many diseases remained beyond the understanding of medical practitioners. Where no test or investigation had been developed to accurately identify that true illness existed, the condition was sometimes diagnosed as hysteria, particularly in women. Here we discuss the case of a 17 year old girl with pain and stiffness in her shoulder. The medical records from the Westminster Hospital have been preserved in the Imperial College London Pathology Museum. They describe how it was initially believed that this teenage girl was not moving her shoulder as a result of suffering from hysteria, rather than due to a genuine musculoskeletal condition affecting the joint. However, with the discovery of X-rays and the subsequent incorporation of radiography into London hospitals in the 1890s, the girl's shoulder was later imaged. This investigation showed the destructive changes of tuberculosis resulting in her undergoing surgery to excise the damaged shoulder joint. The bony changes to the pathological humeral head are described in order to better understand the effects of the TB. Further research revealed information on the surgeon who undertook the operation on this girl, Charles Stonham. Medical texts detailed the hospital management of TB at the time and encapsulate views on treatment options for so called 'hysterical' young women throughout the Victorian era.

Keywords: tuberculosis, hysteria, Victorian period, X-rays, misdiagnosis

Introduction

The aim of this research is to investigate the case of a 17 year old girl who was misdiagnosed with *hysteria* in London during the late Victorian period. The teenage girl was actually suffering from tuberculosis of the shoulder joint, which was only discovered by the Victorians later following access to radiography. The primary source in this case is the excised head of humerus itself - a pathological specimen, which to our knowledge has not been previously published. Viewed in context, we aim to provide an invaluable insight into the disturbing treatment of these girls upon being branded 'hysterical', and also the significance of radiographs in freeing many from this undesirable misdiagnosis.

Hysteria, although not a new concept in the Victorian era continued to be a poorly understood and managed ailment, and one belonging more often than not to women. The definition gradually changed over the course of the nineteenth century initially requiring 'a sort of attack of laughter or sobbing producing very energetic involuntary movements' (Carter, 1853: 2). By the late Victorian period however, no dramatic outburst was necessary and this definition shifted to include a much wider range of phenomena such as 'loss of sensation...nausea, headaches, pain in breast...knee...and spine, as well as paralysis of virtually any extremity (Smith-Rosenberg, 1985: 202). The condition therefore took on a more mimetic quality (Perna, 2004: 12) being seen less as an acute 'fit' and

more as a general collection of many, often vague symptoms. In this way it became something of a medical scapegoat for disorders that until the introduction of new technology were simply undiagnosed or poorly understood.

This slow transformation in beliefs about hysteria also applied to its suspected aetiological factors. Early beliefs were that the condition arose as a result of character weaknesses such as 'a habitual want of self control and a fickle oversensitive character,' largely seen as female traits (Prichard, 1835: 25). By the mid-Victorian era the concept of a nervous cause began to emerge. However, despite this believed organic aetiology, physicians still agreed that the best management of hysteria was in fact using moral treatment or remedial means, even as late as 1900.

Materials

The palaeopathological evidence presented in this study is principally derived from a skeletal specimen currently held in the Imperial College London Pathology Museum, at Charing Cross Hospital. The museum card accompanying the specimen is the old style card, known to have been discontinued in 1900. The card is therefore itself a valuable source since it dates back to the end of the Victorian era (Specimen Card Number W0709). The bone is the head of a left humerus and is well preserved as part of a skeletal collection belonging to the old Westminster Hospital. It was obtained from surgical

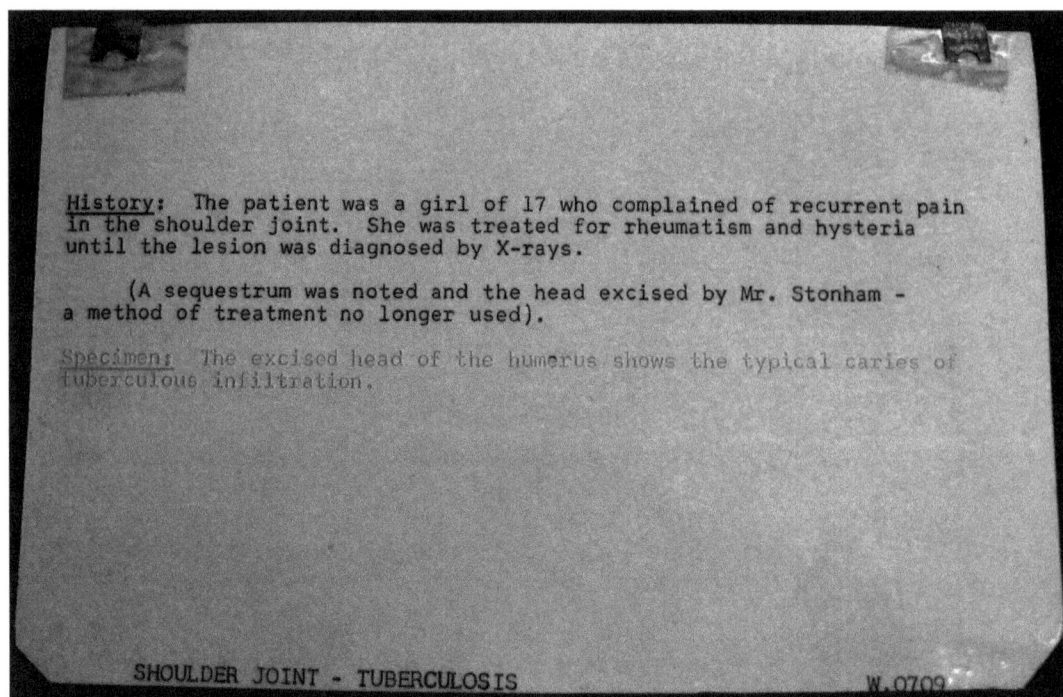

Figure 1. Museum card for specimen W0709, dating from the 1890s.

excision in the late Victorian period. The origin of the specimen is well recorded and the individual was a Londoner, however the Victorian radiograph is not present with the specimen. A recent X-ray of the bone has not been taken in this case.

The main textual evidence for the treatment of this girl comes from the museum card accompanying the specimen. This useful primary source dates back to the time when the bone was acquired. It gives details of her age, symptoms and treatment history. Further primary written evidence includes Victorian texts on medicine, surgery and hysteria. Secondary source written evidence includes modern historical texts on hysteria and women in both early and late Victorian Britain, as well as texts on tuberculosis and X-rays in hospitals. With regards to the girl in this case, no further information regarding her long term follow up or ultimate place or cause of death remains with the specimen. However accounts of the Westminster Hospital, medical journals and a textbook written by the surgeon himself have provided crucial information on Mr Stonham who is known to have excised the bone.

Results

Skeletal pathology

The skeletal specimen was donated to the museum prior to 1900, as the details are recorded on an old-style record card (Fig. 1) that was discontinued by the museum in that year. It was comprised of the head of a left humerus with a very small section of the shaft. The distal part of the specimen had an unnaturally straight edge with no remodelling, thus appearing to have been cut cleanly. This is compatible with the card description which states

that the bone was surgically excised. The lesions seen on the bone were typical of tuberculosis. There was extensive destruction to the articular surface with loss of the smooth subchondral bone. The underlying cancellous bone of the humeral head was clearly visible (Fig. 2). The greater tuberosity was largely destroyed. There was minimal new bone formation, principally at the greater and lesser tuberosities (Fig. 3). This is typical of TB lesions known for being predominantly lytic with minimal new bone formation. (Roberts and Manchester, 2005: 70).

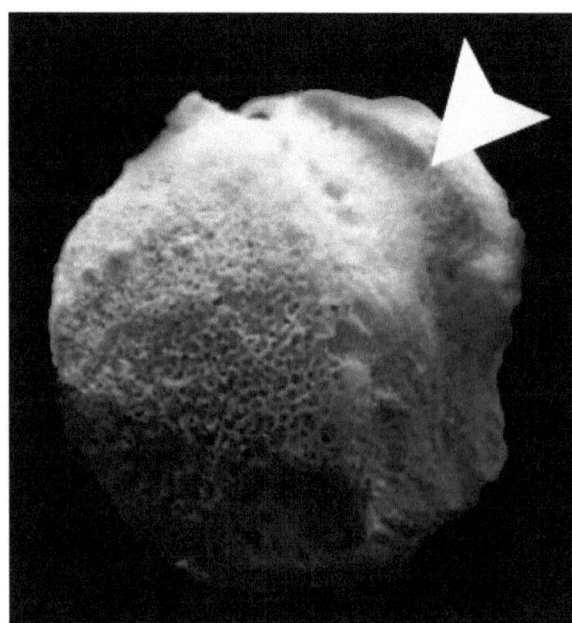

Figure 2. Medial aspect of humeral head showing marked destruction of subchondral bone and negligible new bone formation. Arrow marks greater tuberosity.

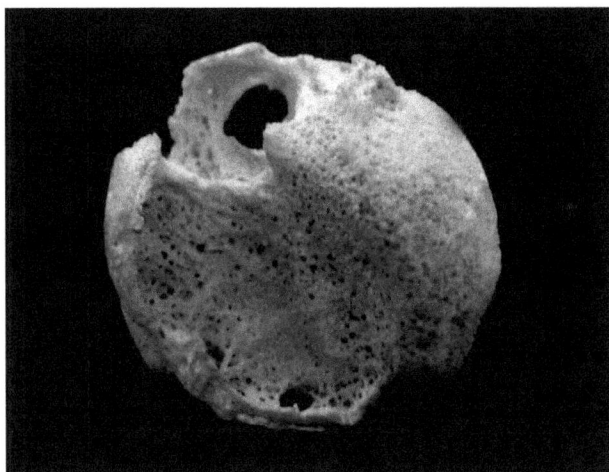

Figure 3. Superior aspect of humeral head showing destructive process. Articular surface lies to the right.

The textual evidence

The museum card was held in the Charing Cross Hospital Pathology Museum and stated that the specimen belonged to a '17 year old girl who complained of recurrent pain in the shoulder' (Fig. 1). The patient was originally treated for hysteria 'until the lesion was diagnosed by X-rays'. She then underwent surgery by a Mr Stonham to excise the humeral head. The card therefore provided verification of the authenticity of the specimen as well as information on the initial misdiagnosis of hysteria which was tentatively changed to TB by the Victorians following the X-ray. This was then confirmed definitively from the histopathology of the surgically excised joint, again by the Victorians, when it was removed. They then entered the specimen into the pathology museum as a clearly diagnosed case of joint TB. Overall therefore, these vital clues from the card including the date, origin of the specimen and the surgeon's name, all created an excellent starting point for further research.

Discussion

This young woman suffered with tuberculosis of the shoulder, which initially was not identified. As such the symptoms and signs of the disease were interpreted by clinicians of the day to represent a case of hysteria. The museum card does not record the treatment given to this girl prior to her surgery, but a number of options are recorded in texts from the period. The British Physician Carter advocated 'observant neglect' for hysteria in which 'indifference to the patient's expectations of sympathy' (Carter, 1853: 109) was enacted to establish the physician's lofty authority. His clinical textbook on hysteria also encouraged making the patient admit 'moral wretchedness and confess sins' in order to combat their 'weak needy character and sexual repression' (Carter, 1853: 109). Another popular textbook among physicians and surgeons in the late Victorian era was American, S.W. Mitchell's (1877) publication: *Fat and blood: and*

how to make them. This took a physical rather than psychological approach. He believed the root of hysteria to be the pressure on women "to lose weight and have figures like little boys" so the cure in his eyes was to fatten them up with high calorie-intake diets (Mitchell, 1877: 27).

In terms of hysteria linked to pain in the limbs (as in this teenage case), the early Victorian physician Hall recommended exercise for the 'idle' middle class women. He was prone to prescribing that 'one should walk to the serpentine and dip one's finger in it' (Hall, 1836: 130) simply as a way of getting women in London to stretch their legs. In terms of pharmacological treatment, it was common in the nineteenth century to prescribe zinc, or potassium bromide and cod liver oil as general treatments for these girls (Tanner, 1891: 155). However as hysteria became an increasingly common diagnosis it was seen as a hugely lucrative area for drug companies and patents for drugs such as 'pectoral drops' rapidly emerged:

> "Pectoral drops... a new chymicall peparacon ...antihysterick, working chiefly by sweat and urine, exceeding all other medicines yet found out for rheumatism...agues and hystericks" (Okell, 1857: 1).

Closer to the end of the century was the arrival of "Elixir Godineau" (Godineau, 1895), which, like pectoral drops may well have been one of the treatments taken by the patient in this case. The advertising booklet gives descriptions of patient success stories such as:

> "Miss D. 30yrs of age had hysteria...bromides did not improve her condition then she tried Elixir Godineau...the patient may now be looked upon as cured" (Godineau, 1895: 52).

On the whole, treatments were aimed at various aspects of the patient's lifestyle, from pharmacological drugs including "vast quantities of alcohol and opium based palliatives" (Jordan, 1993: 26) sold at local dispensaries to moral remedies or recommendations for exercise such as gymnastics and walking (Tanner, 1891: 155). Treatments varied greatly both in severity and effectiveness, which is arguably unsurprising given that diagnoses of hysteria were incorrect. The likely range of conditions misdiagnosed in this way would completely negate the possibility of finding a remedy that worked universally amongst these patients.

The large variation in treatment ideas most likely stems from the wide range of causation theories for hysteria at the time. Hall believed that women "possessed a greater blood capillary density" than men- based on female menstruation (Hall, 1836:130). He linked this to greater susceptibility of the nervous system than is observed in males and labelled hysteria *'mimosis Urens'* also linking the condition with lack of a varied diet causing constipation. "A woman's tendency to delay in yielding to the first solicitations of nature to evacuate the bowels" (Hall, 1836: 130) was in his eyes the physical root of the problem. The French Physician Louyer-Villermay concurred that the physical cause was "voluntary and forced continence" as well as "an ardent and lascivious uterine system" (Louyer-Villermay, 1816: 232). In terms of the *mental* and *lifestyle* aetiological factors, Villermay included:

> "a burning imagination... an overly tender heart...prolonged exposure to sunrays or cold... over use of perfumes...truffles, vanilla ...too long a stay in bed, and the reading of novels" (Louyer-Villermay, 1816: 232-233).

Alternative views on the physiological cause of hysteria included that of Scottish Physician William Cullen who described "diminished or increased nervous system excitability producing spasmodic or atonic symptoms" (Cullen, 1796: 49). Also, Paris physician Landouzy known for his particularly harsh view described "the female genital apparatus as the unique seat of hysteria" (Landouzy, 1846: 211). More than most he saw the uterine system as the source and his theory received extremely strong support well into the mid-nineteenth century (Beizer, 1994: 36).

The discovery of X-rays in 1895 by Roentgen, a physicist and professor at the Physical Institute of Wurzburg (Williams, 1982: 361) was followed very swiftly by attempts to apply this technology to medicine. Almost simultaneously in 1896 A.H. Becquerel discovered uranium, then in 1898 the Curies discovered radium (Williams, 1982: 362). These developments triggered the establishment of a series of companies competing to produce photographic plates in London (Burrows, 1986: 62). Although permanent X-ray units were installed almost immediately (in 1896) in the most famous hospitals such as Guys and St Thomas's, records show that Westminster where the teenage girl was treated was not one of the first (Burrows, 1986: 76). By 1907 however Westminster had a thriving Department of Electrotherapy and Radiography so at some point between these two dates the use of this technology became an integral part of the diagnostic process. To put this into context, the London hospitals were not the only sites to hold such technology and smaller hospitals outside the capital were anxious to have the benefits of the new tool (Pickstone, 1985: 199). Liverpool infirmary set up a radiographic service in 1896 and in Manchester a firm of pharmacists built up a large private practice taking X-radiographs for Manchester practitioners' (Pickstone, 1985: 199). The girl at Westminster clearly had an image taken of her shoulder prior to 1900, as this triggered her operation. However with radiography in it's early stages it must be noted that radiologists were constantly wrestling with inefficient apparatus (Holland, 1916: 350). As such, radiography use was limited where possible to simple parts of the body such as the peripheries, whereas chest and abdominal X-rays were not introduced until shortly after World War One (Bynum, 1994: 175).

The capacity of this technology for increased diagnostic accuracy created huge excitement amongst physicians and surgeons who set up special societies and journals to discuss and develop X-ray techniques (Dibner, 1962: 37). However, it must be recognised that radiography was not received gratefully by all (Doby and Alker, 1997: 64). Many saw it as a tool for those in power to further assert themselves through making medicine increasingly scientific and claiming special expertise (Howell, 1995: 158). Moreover exposure and clarity of image could often be disappointing. Victorian physician Shenton, in an actual case of joint TB wrote:

> "It is a rule and a good rule to bear in mind...that radiograms of tubercular disease in bones and joints are always disappointing from a pictorial point of view" (Shenton, 1911: 143).

The above source, although possibly not representative of all physicians is suggestive of the potential for poor image quality. On the whole therefore it must be noted that although it did have limits, fortunately for many women radiography made hysteria a less acceptable blanket explanation for physicians, in time becoming "something of an invaluable adjunct in diagnosis" (Pullin, and Wiltshire 1927). In a broader context however, the X-ray machine was an innovation that came to carry huge symbolic power. Although initially some were sceptical and "relegated the technology to an obscure corner", it slowly emerged to typify the ultimate "go-ahead hospital" (Stanton, 1999: 439).

In terms of managing joint TB, Victorian medical textbooks illustrate that 'distraction' or 'extension of the joint' was a common hospital treatment. This was achieved using weights and a pulley to stretch the arm (Fig. 4). Distraction was often accompanied by massage or tapping of the joint with a needle and syringe to alleviate stiffness.

Since the tuberculin vaccine was still in it's animal experimentation stage in the 1880s and Koch's ideas on the contagiousness of tuberculosis were not widely disseminated or accepted in Britain until the late 1890s (Pickstone, 1992: 49) most treatments were mild conservative measures. These included "sea bathing and change of climate" or drugs such as "potassium iodide...as it retards the development and reproduction of the bacillus" (Cheyne, 1911: 325). However hospital treatment prior to surgery for the 17-year-old girl could have consisted of anything from simple immobilisation of the shoulder with a sling to cautery or parenchymatous injections with iodoform (Jones, 1887: 183). Ultimately it appears that surgery was the most promising option for the girl and since long anterior excisions became increasingly popular from the 1870s prompted by the discovery of the complete mechanics of the shoulder at this time (Le Vay, 1956: 41) it is no surprise that this was the operation chosen for her.

The museum card accompanying the specimen names Mr Stonham as the surgeon who operated on the girl. In search for some biographical details such as his

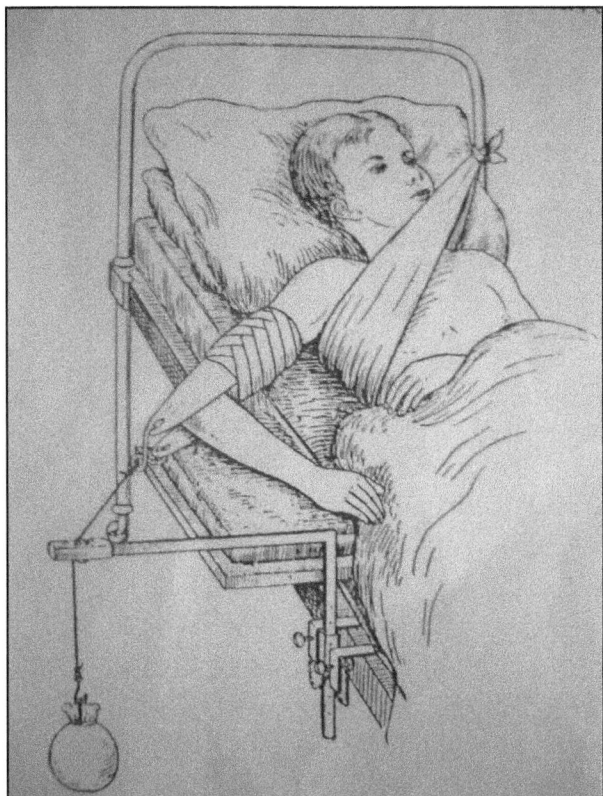

Figure 4. Traction for disease of the shoulder joint in a publication of 1911 (Cheyne, 1911, 324). Reproduced with permission of Oxford University Press.

background, education that he had and whether his practises were common at the time; it soon became apparent that Mr Stonham had been a very prominent figure in the surgical field. He wrote an extensive *Manual of Surgery* in three volumes published in 1899, which details all the common surgical conditions and operative procedures for both general and regional surgery (Stonham, 1899). Other clues suggestive of Mr Stonham's importance in the field are that two prominent medical journals, *the Lancet* and the *British Medical Journal* (*BMJ*) dedicate over a page to his obituary in the year of his death (1916) recounting details of his life and praising his work.

Originally Mr Stonham (1858-1916) was born in Maidstone, Kent and was educated at King's School in Canterbury before attending University College London to study Medicine. He graduated from there as a Gold medallist in Surgery, Medicine and Gynaecology and went on to hold resident posts at the hospital (Obituary, *BMJ* 1916). This information alone suggests that Charles Stonham was clearly an extremely promising student and probably one of the best in his year. He took his MRCS and became a fellow of the Royal College of Surgeons in 1884 then assisted as a demonstrator at the University College Pathology museum before being given the post of assistant surgeon at Westminster Hospital in 1887 (Obituary, *BMJ* 1916). He remained at this hospital to be appointed full surgeon in 1895 and Senior surgeon in 1897. During his career he was also a lecturer and examiner at various universities, wrote a surgical

textbook, and was asked to contribute to medical dictionaries on various topics (Obituary, *the Lancet* 1916). His colleague at Westminster Mr Walter G. Spencer describes Stonham as:

> "perfectly ambidextrous...his long thin hands were used most skilfully...he will be remembered at Westminster for many brilliant successes and for many acts of kindness to patients, students and nurses" (Obituary, *BMJ* 1916).

Records of the Westminster Hospital describe Charles Stonham as someone who eagerly seized on the new principles of Lister and was "revivifying the practices and teachings of surgery in a remarkable manner" (Humble, 1966: 156). Around the time of admittance of the 17-year old, sources show that the hospital had been newly reconstructed with a clinical lab building, hence culture of the TB bacillus would have been possible. Also new technology and diagnostic techniques would have become available with this modernisation, improving accuracy as in our case.

It can be deduced then that since Mr Stonham was the main surgeon in the operation for excision of our specimen, that this surgery took place after 1896 when he was appointed to this position. In 1901 Stonham was described as having "formed the Imperial Yeomannery Field Hospital and Bearer Company and in the Spring set sail for the South African War" (Humble, 1966: 160). On his return, Mr Stonham turned his hand to organising the Mounted Brigade Field Ambulance (Langdon-Davies, 1952: 42) he was mobilised with it and in June 1915 was appointed Consulting Surgeon to the forces in Egypt with the rank of Full Colonel (Obituary, *BMJ* 1916). This suggests that the operation on the teenage girl must have taken place before this, while he still worked at Westminster as a Senior Surgeon (between 1896 and 1901). This is confirmed by the fact that Stonham did not return to the hospital after the war as sadly whilst serving in Egypt he contracted Dengue fever and: "prostrate by dengue had to return home on sick leave. His illness proved to be fatal on January 31st 1916" (Obituary, *BMJ* 1916: 258).

This information on Stonham's life and career helps put his work into context and illustrates that amongst surgeons in the late Victorian era, Stonham was both renowned and respected. However, looking more specifically at his manual of surgery (Stonham, 1899) it is interesting to note what he personally believed constituted hysteria and tuberculosis and how best to manage these two conditions relevant to the case at hand. Volume 2 of the manual entitled "Injuries" includes a section on hysteria which Stonham subdivides into: Acute cases where the patient "may exhibit emotional symptoms such as laughing or sobbing" and Chronic hysteria which may involve long periods of "paralysis...anaesthesias...and melancholia" (Stonham, 1899: 262). This seems more likely to be the type diagnosed in the girl with longstanding pain and inability to optimally move her shoulder. He described "mental anxiety" as a powerful cause and believed the best treatment to be removing the patient from friends and family and placing them with strangers with strictly minimal bed rest so as not to enhance their misconception that the paralysis was due to "organic mischief" (Stonham, 1899: 269). He also strongly advocated "massage...cold douching, plenty of food and bromide of ammonia" (Stonham, 1899: 269).

For joint TB however, although he includes specific sections on the hip, knee, elbow and sacroiliac joints there is not one for the shoulder suggesting that the site of the disease in this case is probably quite rare. In his general description of joint TB he refers to it as a disease of early life and the poorer classes, (Stonham, 1899: 160) which could tell us something about the girl's lifestyle. Also he recommends sodium chloride solution to 'diminish the vascularity' and weight extension (Fig. 1) as treatments of mild to moderate disease (Stonham, 1899: 160). He reserved surgery for:

> "more advanced cases where the bones are extensively involved, the ligaments are softened and destroyed, where the sinuses extend among the periarticular structures" (Stonham, 1899: 161).

The girl in our case must therefore have had this very advanced form of the disease. He described the two main surgical options in this extreme case as complete excision (which is the preferred option if the circumstances permit) or as a final resort – amputation (Stonham, 1899: 161).

On the whole, being a senior surgeon and having published a manual of surgery around the time of the shoulder excision operation, his methods were clearly typical of surgery in the late Victorian period and probably at the cutting edge of it. The level of care that the girl received can therefore safely be assumed to have been among the best available at the time.

Conclusion

Overall, the case of the 17 year old girl has proved extremely enlightening in illustrating not only how a young girl branded as 'hysterical' would have been treated in the Victorian era but also how attitudes to the disease evolved over the course of the century. Furthermore researching this thesis has brought to light new evidence of consequences that arose from such a misdiagnosis, as a result of the treatments inflicted on these girls. Prior to radiography she may have spent years with disability and discomfort as the infection progressed. The introduction of X-ray technology was, although not an instant revolution as some accounts suggest, vital in improving detection of numerous conditions. In particular TB lesions in the limbs were sometimes visible on X-ray, diminishing the number of physicians who in their ignorance were referring to the highly convenient alternative of 'hysteria' in women. It would be naive, however to think that the trend of diagnosing numerous ailments as hysteria simply vanished with the early onset

of X-rays. This in fact ultimately took several decades, not disappearing largely until after World War One, following further technological advances. The case of the girl treated at Westminster therefore does not merely highlight the possibility that TB was mistaken for hysteria, but also that many diseases were poorly understood at the time. X-rays therefore made a key contribution to identifying a range of diseases including tuberculosis.

Acknowledgements

We are grateful for the assistance of Dr. Vin Chauhan, curator of the Charing Cross Hospital Pathology Museum.

Literature Cited

Beizer, J. 1994. *Ventriloquized Bodies: Narratives of Hysteria in Nineteenth-Century France*. Ithaca: Cornell University Press:

Burrows, E.H. 1986. *Pioneers and Early Years: A History of British Radiology*. Channel Islands: Colophon Ltd.

Bynum, W.F. 1994. *Science and the Practice of Medicine in the Nineteenth Century*. Cambridge: Cambridge University Press.

Carter, R.B. 1853. *On the Pathology and Treatment of Hysteria*. London: John Churchill.

Cheyne, Sir. W.W. 1911. *Tuberculous Diseases of Bones and Joints, their Pathology, Symptoms, and Treatment*. Second Edition. London: Henry Frowde.

Cullen, W. 1796. *First Lines of the Practice of Physic with Practical and Explanatory Notes by John Rotherham*. Edinburgh: Bell & Badfute.

Dibner, B. 1962. *The New Rays of Professor Roentgen*. Norwalk: Burndy Library Inc.

Doby, T. and Alker, G. 1997. *Origins and Developments of Medical Imaging*. Carbondale: Southern Illinois University Press.

Godineau, L. 1895. *'Extension of Life' by Elixir Godineau*. Paris: publisher not stated.

Hall, M 1836. *Lectures on the Nervous System and its Diseases*. London: Sherwood, Gilbert and Piper.

Holland, C.T. 1916. "Presidential address to the Roentgen Society". *Archives of Radiology and Electrotherapy* 21: 347-403.

Howell, J.D. 1995. *Technology in the Hospital-Transforming Patient Care in the Early Twentieth Century.* Baltimore: John Hopkins University Press.

Humble, J.G. 1966 "Westminster Hospital: The first 250 years" *British Medical Journal* 1: 5480:156-162.

Jones, T. 1887. *Diseases of the Bones.* London: Smith Elder & Co.

Jordan, T. E. 1993. *The Degeneracy Crisis and Victorian Youth.* Albany: State University of New York Press.

Landouzy, M. H. 1846. *Traité complet de l'hysterie.* Paris: Balliere.

Langdon-Davies, J. 1952. *Westminster Hospital: Two Centuries of Voluntary Service 1719-1948.* London: John Murray Ltd.

Le Vay, D. 1956. *The life of Hugh Owen Thomas.* Edinburgh: Livingstone.

Louyer-Villermay, J. B. 1816. *Traité des Maladies Nerveuses ou Vapeurs : et particulièrement de l'hystérie et de l'hypocondrie.* Paris: Chez Méquignon l'ainé père.

Mitchell, S.W. 1877. *Fat and Blood; and How to Make Them.* Philadelphia: J.B. Lippincott and Co.

Museum Specimen Card number W0709, Imperial College Pathology Museum, Charing Cross Hospital, London.

"Obituary". 1916. *British Medical Journal* 1:258.

"Obituary". 1916. *Lancet* 1:375-376.

Okell, B. 1857. "Patent for 'Pectoral drops" *Patents and Specifications; Medical and Surgical 1698-1858.* London: Great Seal Patent Office, Holborn, Vol .1362:1

Perna, S.F. 2004. "The function and diagnosis of hysteria in nineteenth century fiction and medical texts." Dissertation: Ann Arbor: UMI dissertation services, University Microfilms International.

Pickstone, J. V. 1985 *Medicine and Industrial Society: A History of Hospital Development in Manchester and its Region 1752-1946.* Manchester: Manchester University.

Pickstone, J. V. 1992 (ed.) *Medical Innovations in Historical Perspective.* Basingstoke: Macmillan.

Prichard, J.C. 1835. *A Treatise on Insanity and Other Disorders Affecting the Mind.* London: Hunter and MacAlpine.

Pullin, V.E.A. and Wiltshire, W.J. 1927. *X-rays Past and Present.* London: Ernest-Benn Ltd.

Roberts, C.A. and Manchester, K. 2005. *The Archaeology of Disease.* Stroud: Sutton Publishing.

Shenton, E.W.H. 1911. *Disease in the Bone and its Detection by the X-rays.* London: Macmillan.

Smith-Rosenberg, C. 1985. *Disorderly Conduct: Visions of Gender in Victorian America.* New York: A.A. Knopf.

Stanton, J. 1999. "Making Sense of Technologies in Medicine" *Social History of Medicine* 12: 4437-448.

Stonham, C. 1899. *A Manual of Surgery.* London: Macmillan.

Tanner, T.H. 1891. *Index of Diseases and Their Treatment.* London: Henry Renshaw.

Williams, T.I. 1982. *A Short History of Twentieth Century Technology ca 1900-ca 1950.* Oxford: Clarendon Press.

External auditory exostosis "at the end of the world": the southernmost evidence according to the latitudinal hypothesis

Paola Ponce[1*], Gabriela Ghidini[2], Rolando González-José[3]

[1] Department of Archaeology, University of Durham, Durham DH1 3LE, England.
[2] Departamento Científico de Antropología, Facultad de Ciencias Naturales y Museo, Universidad Nacional de La Plata, Buenos Aires, Argentina.
[3] Centro Nacional Patagónico, Consejo Nacional de Investigaciones Científicas y Técnicas. Puerto Madryn, Argentina.
*e-mail address for correspondence: p.v.ponce@durham.ac.uk

Abstract

External auditory exostoses (EAE) are bony anomalies of the external auricular canal associated with prolonged exposure to cold water. According to the latitudinal hypothesis proposed by Kennedy (1986), its prevalence falls as the latitude increases north and south above 45°, due to the risk of hypothermia from swimming in cold waters. The aim of this paper was to examine the evidence for EAE in the southernmost ethnographic groups who ever inhabited the world. For this purpose, 108 crania of adult males and females housed at different museums were used. They belonged to Amerindians from Tierra del Fuego who practised two different life strategies, a terrestrial hunting-gathering economy and an adaptation to marine resources. Six crania exhibited EAE (5.5%) from which only one was male (0.9%) and five were females (4.6%). Five out of 55 crania (9.1%) whose subsistence economy was mainly based on marine products exhibited EAE. On the other hand, among those whose diet was primarily based on terrestrial resources, the prevalence was 1.9% (one out of 53 crania had EAE). Although the prevalence difference between both groups was not statistically significant (p>0.05), these results suggest that EAE might be associated with exposure to cold water due to exploitation of marine resources although further investigations are necessary to confirm this hypothesis. In accordance with Kennedy's hypothesis the frequency of EAE was low, as expected in such a hostile and harsh cold environment.

Keywords: auricular exostosis, hunter-gatherers, Amerindians, Tierra del Fuego

Introduction

External auditory exostoses (EAE) have also been called "aural exostosis" (Roche, 1964), "auditory torus" (Berry and Berry, 1967; Brothwell, 1981), "torus acusticus", "torus tympanicus", "torus auditivus" (Hauser and De Stefano, 1989: 186) and "bony outgrowths" (Karegeannes, 1995). In the clinical literature and due to the high frequency of EAE amongst those engaged in aquatic sports, it has also been called "surfer's ear" or "diver's ear" (Seftel, 1977; Ikeda, 1998; Kroon et al., 2002).

External auditory exostoses are benign bony anomalies of variable size and number commonly found unilaterally or bilaterally in the outer walls of the external auditory canal. Microscopically, they are comprised of dense layers of subperiosteal compact bone (Graham, 1979; Hutchinson et al., 1997) and covered with normal epithelium in the patient. Although its presence is non-symptomatic, secondary effects of ear canal occlusion are very common. For instance, it has been reported that tinnitus (ringing sound in the ear), hearing loss or recurrent otitis externa (Timofeev et al., 2004) as well as infection due to cerumen blockage (DiBartolomeo, 1979; Kroon et al., 2002) are among the commonest complications cited by the clinicians. The use of earplugs can prevent the development of EAE and its side effects (DiBartolomeo, 1979). However, if no form of prevention is taken and the occlusion progresses, then a surgical removal may be necessary.

The two dominant yet contradictory hypotheses that have tried to explain the etiological factors that trigger the development of EAE are genetic-hereditary and exposure to cold water. The former has been postulated by Berry and Berry (1967) and subsequently applied to a large number of anthropological cases to measure biodistances between prehistoric populations. Examples of this kind are Ossenberg (1976), Perizonius (1979) and Hanihara et al. (2003). On the other hand, the latter has been more widely accepted by clinicians (Karegeannes, 1995; Deleyiannis et al., 1996; Ikeda, 1998; Kroon et al., 2002; Altuna Mariezkurrena et al., 2004; Timofeev et al., 2004) and supported experimentally (Fowler and Osmun, 1942) as an activity-induced pathology. Several studies carried out in the anthropological field have also supported this hypothesis (Frayer, 1988; Manzi et al., 1991; Standen et al., 1997; Velasco-Vazquez et al., 2000; Arnay-de-la-Rosa et al., 2001). However, recent studies (Hutchinson et al., 1997) have questioned the cold-water hypothesis as the unique factor responsible for the EAE presence.

In essence, the cold-water hypothesis suggests that prolonged immersion in cold water produces periosteal sensitivity and irritation of the ear canal in people who engage in water sports such as divers and surfers (Altuna Mariezkurrena et al., 2004) or people who exploit marine or freshwater resources (Kennedy, 1986). This in turn triggers focal osteoblastic activity that leads to a bony formation or exostosis (Timofeev *et al.*, 2004).

In 1986, Kennedy carried out a thorough study and recorded the presence of EAE according to latitude. She found that the lowest frequencies (<5%) were observed in polar and sub polar areas (above 45° N and below 45° S) where the risk of hypothermia would have prevented people from fully immersing themselves in the search for marine resources. Comparatively, those who lived in tropical latitudes (between 0° - 30° N and S) would have had a low probability of developing auditory exostosis, as the water temperatures would not be sufficiently cold to produce the anomaly. In contrast, higher frequencies (>21%) were found in subtropical latitudes (between 30° - 45° N and S) where access to marine and fresh water resources would have encouraged people to swim in tepid or mild temperatures (15°C - 19°C) and be prone to develop EAE. According to Kennedy (1986:408) "no data on auditory exostoses were found for populations living beyond 45° south latitude". Therefore the objective of this paper, after considering Kennedy's latitudinal analysis of the occurrence of EAE, is to test its presence in the southernmost archaeological populations who ever inhabited the southern hemisphere and one of the world's harshest environments and ultimately to test its relationship with the cold-water aetiology.

Environmental considerations

The island of Tierra del Fuego is located at the southernmost part of Argentina and Chile and has been divided between both countries since 1881 (García-Moro *et al.*, 1997). The island is the southernmost inhabited land in the world. Geographically it is located between 52° 27′ north and 55° 59′ south and has an extension of 40,000 km². Its extreme southern location and its proximity to Antarctica are significant determinant factors of the environmental conditions and climate whose temperatures range from 27° C in summer to minus 20° C in winter. The duration of daylight hours is also strikingly contrasting. During winter there are only 6 hours compared to 20 hours of daylight in summer (García-Moro *et al.*, 1997).

Given that water temperature has been widely recognised as a detrimental factor in the aetiology of EAE, the surface water temperature in the Ushuaia Station near the Beagle channel was obtained. Table 1 shows the average seawater temperature throughout the year during the period 1984-1996 taken by the Centro Multidisciplinario de Investigaciones Científicas of Tierra del Fuego (CADIC).

The annual average temperature of the superficial seawater is 6.3°C, which would be more than sufficiently cold to produce EAE in people that dive on a prolonged basis and for a number of years. For instance, it has been demonstrated clinically that EAE can increase in size as well as in prevalence with age depending on the time spent in the water, the frequency of immersion and the

season of the year. The majority of the clinicians consider that the "cut-off point" temperature to produce EAE ranges between 10°C-15°C (Deleyiannis, 1996; Kroon *et al.*, 2002). However, in regard of the number of years necessary to obstruct the ear canal there is little agreement. It has been suggested that obstruction can occur in as little as three years (Karegeannes, 1995), five years or less (Deleyiannis *et al.*, 1996), and a median of seven years (Kroon *et al.*, 2002) and a cut-off point of ten to 12 years (DiBartolomeo, 1979; Altuna Mariezkurrena *et al.*, 2004) are necessary.

Table 1. Mean values for surface sea temperatures in the Beagle Channel. From Orquera and Piana (1999).

Month	Temp. ° C
Jan	8.6
Feb	8.6
Mar	7.9
Apr	6.7
May	5.5
Jun	4.7
July	4.3
Aug	1.3
Sept	4.5
Oct	5.4
Nov	6.7
Dec	8

According to Orquera and Piana (1999) the exposure to wind as well as the low temperatures can explain the conditioning climatic situation of Tierra del Fuego. For instance, the average maximum daily wind speed at the Naval Base in Ushuaia during the period of 1971-1980 was 51 km/h. The combined effect of low temperatures and high winds generates extreme wind-chill factors. For example, with winter temperatures of minus 3°C, winds blowing from 20 to 30 km/h and humidity over 90%, the wind-chill factor drops to minus 17°C.

Materials and methods

A total of 108 crania of adult males and females belonging to Amerindians who inhabited the Tierra de Fuego Island (or Great Island) were used for the present study. They were housed at different museums and scientific institutions in Argentina, Chile and Europe (Table 2). The chronological age at which individuals lived was obtained from diverse sources. In some cases it was fairly precise, in other it was only inferred. The archaeologists and explorers of the late 19th and early 20th century that excavated these remains often gave little information regarding the context of the human remains. However, in general terms, it can be said that they all belonged to the Late Holocene period (González-José, 2003).

These "Fuegian" samples belonged to the Selk'nam, Haush, Yamanas and Alacaluf Amerindians. In relation to other inhabited land in the world, these hunter-gatherers were settled at the southernmost latitudinal region (Fig. 1). Selk'nam and Haush were also known as the

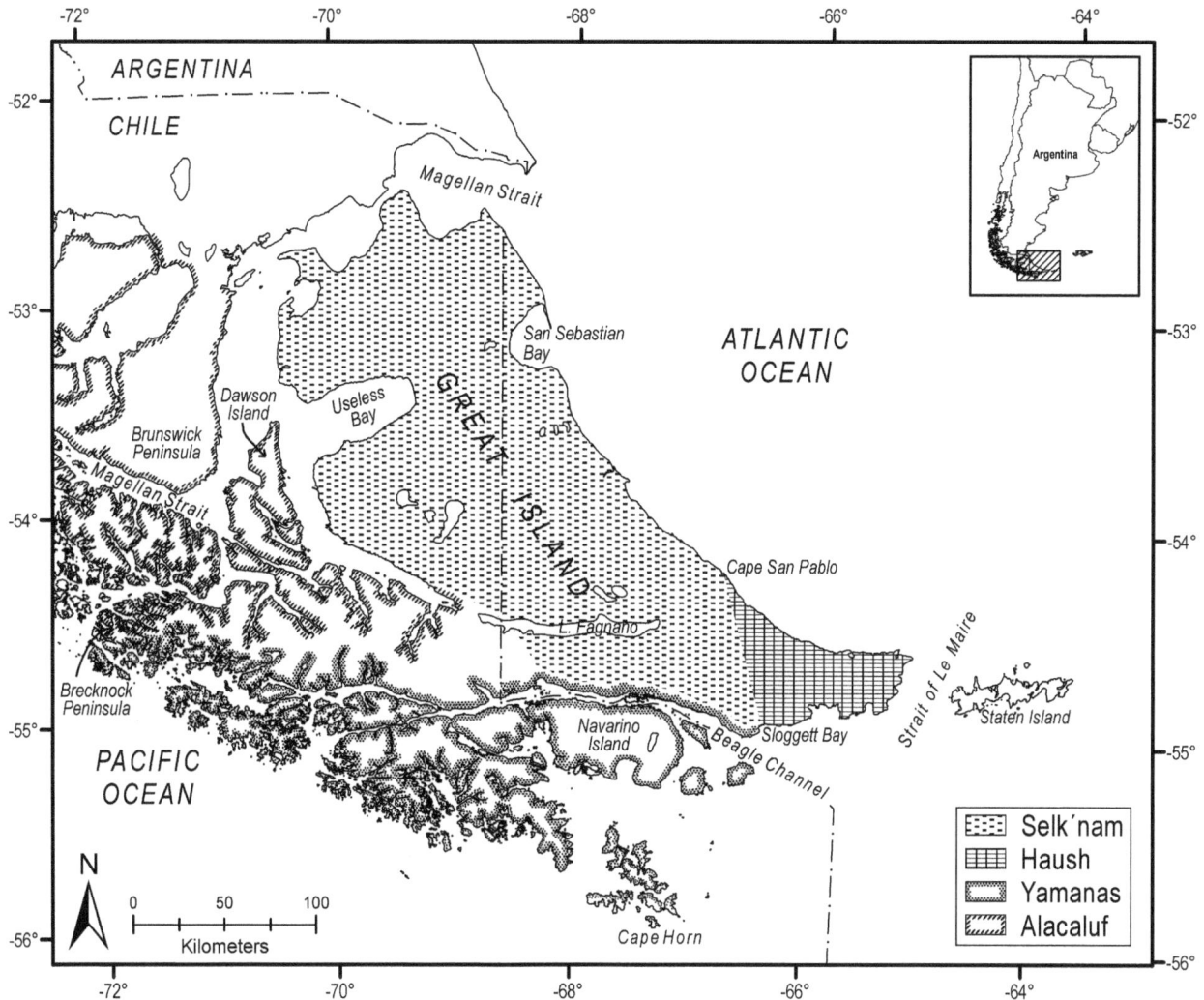

Figure 1. Map of Tierra del Fuego. Modified from Chapman (1986).

"terrestrial nomads" (Chapman, 1986:72-3) because they were settled inland and highly dependent on terrestrial resources such as the guanaco (*Lama guanicoe*), a small American camelid abundant in Tierra del Fuego and the Patagonia. The former group was settled across the whole of Tierra del Fuego Island bordered to the north boundary by the Magellan straits and to the south by the Andean Mountains. The Haush lived in the extreme southeast region of the Tierra del Fuego island and were closely related with the Selk'nams to the point that some authors consider them as the "southern Selk'nams" (Gusinde, 1937, 1979). Their territory encompassed cape San Pablo over the Atlantic coast and the Sloggett bay on the opposite side of the island and the Beagle channel coast.

Both groups shared a similar subsistence economy complementing their diet by hunting, foxes, rodents and birds with bow and arrows; an activity that was restricted to men. Women were in charge of collecting wild mushrooms, berries and other vegetables as well as the systematic gathering of seafood such as mussels, limpets, clams and sea snails. Men helped occasionally in these tasks by employing fishing nets and building small dams in the rivers (Chapman, 1986:46-7). According to

Massone and Prieto (2005) the exceptional event of stranded whales on the seashore was a significant event in the life of this people, as they did not develop any strategy of hunting them nor were able to sail. The whale meat and its fat were of particular importance during the winter and the beginning of the spring when the meat of guanaco was lean.

Yamanas and Alacalufs were the western neighbours of the Selk'nam and Haush. The former group inhabited the southernmost part of the Andean Mountains, from the Southeast coast of the Tierra del Fuego Island and the Brecknock peninsula to the islands around the Cape Horn. The latter group lived in the vast region of the archipelago that today belongs to Chile, near the Brecknock peninsula in the south and Las Peñas gulf in the north.

Both "marine nomads" shared similar subsistence economies, which according to Gusinde (1961) was advantageous when compared with their terrestrial counterparts as the sea offered more generous products than the interior. Women contributed enormously to the economy of the family by fishing and gathering shellfish.

These activities were particularly important; especially when the animals hunted by men were scarce. For this purpose, women used fishing lines and rowed canoes, and occasionally diving down to the sea bottom that was densely strewn with mussels and other marine animals. As the mistress of the canoe, she took her husband to those places where he wanted to try his luck and go after game (Gusinde, 1961). Provided with small harpoons, men were in charge of hunting large marine animals such as seals, sea lions and followed exhausted whales floating-sick in shallow waters (Gusinde, 1961; Massone and Prieto, 2005). They also hunted other mammals such as guanacos, otter and foxes although the last two ones exclusively for their skin. Paleodietary analysis carried out in human bone belonging to these four Amerindian groups also confirms the dietary trend suggested by the ethnohistoric accounts (Borrero *et al.*, 2001; Yesner *et al.*, 2003).

Table 2. Location of the samples.

Institution	No. of skulls
Museo de La Plata (Buenos Aires, Argentina)	6
Museo Etnográfico (Buenos Aires, Argentina)	17
Museo de la Misión Salesiana "La Candelaria" (Rio Grande, Argentina)	11
Instituto de la Patagonia (Punta Arenas, Chile)	23
Museo Regional Maggiorino Borgatello (Punta Arenas, Chile)	14
Museo Regional de Porvenir (Porvenir, Chile)	13
Musee du L'homme (Paris, France)	8
Museo di Antropologia e Etnografia, Instituto di Antropologia (Firenze, Italy)	6
Museum der Anthropologie (Zurich, Switzerland)	3
Natural History Museum (London, England)	7
Total	108

The crania belonging to this set of four Amerindians were grouped according to their geographical origin as "terrestrial" and "marine" Fuegian. Thus, terrestrial Fuegians were those who lived in the interior of Tierra del Fuego and whose subsistence economy was mainly based on hunting guanaco such as the Selk'nam and Haush. Yamanas and Alacalufs were the marine Fuegians who settled in the coastal areas of the island and exploited the resources that the sea offered. González-José *et al.* (2002) and Lalueza *et al.* (1997) previously discussed the genetic relationship and population dynamics among Fuegian groups. Based on a population-genetics study of craniofacial shape (González-José *et al.*, 2002) and from ancient DNA samples from Fuegian and Patagonian Indians, both studies conclude that marine and terrestrial stocks belonged to a single genetic pool,

which occupied the Tierra del Fuego Island prior, the formation of the Magellan Strait.

If Kennedy's hypothesis (1986) were correct, we should expect to find a low prevalence of EAE among these four populations because the cold-water temperatures would have discouraged them from full body immersion and the risk of hypothermia. Furthermore, if the cold-water hypothesis is the best etiological explanation for the presence of EAE, then we should find a higher frequency of EAE among the marine group rather than the terrestrial one.

Sex was assessed considering the dimorphic traits of the skull following the standards proposed by Buikstra and Ubelaker (1994). When the skull did not provide a definite diagnose the pelvis was also used whenever present. The age of the individuals was recorded following the cranial suture closure patterns for age estimation proposed by Buikstra and Ubelaker (1994).

Both ear canals were observed and inspected with the naked eye for the presence of EAE. The prevalence of EAE was assessed by considering affected crania rather than counting the number of temporal bones with the condition. In other words, if the condition was present either unilaterally or bilaterally, then the presence was scored only once.

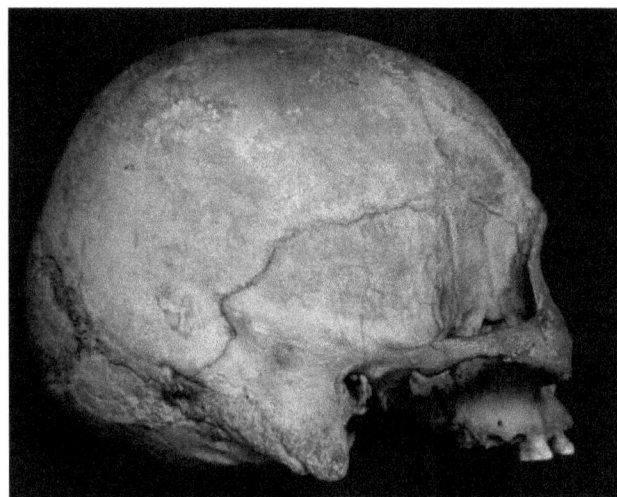

Figure 2. Latero-posterior view of skull 1025.7 from an adult female from Ushuaia (with permission of the Natural History Museum, London).

Results

Sex assessment resulted in 56 males and 52 females. Assessment of provenance was equally split with 55 marine Fuegian versus 53 terrestrial (Table 3). From the total 108 crania studied, six had EAE (5.5%) from which only one was male (0.9%) and the remaining five females (4.6%). The difference in sexual prevalence was not significant ($\chi^2 = 2.6$; $p>0.05$). Individuals with EAE were classified as young adults (n.=1) and middle adults (n.=5).

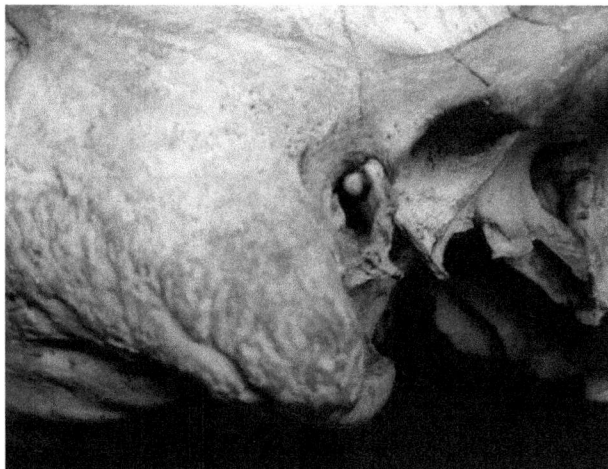

Figure 3. Close view of exostosis at the right external ear canal (with permission of the Natural History Museum, London).

Based on the geographical origin of the Fuegian Amerindians, it was found that five (four females and one male) out of 55 crania (9.1%) whose subsistence economy was mainly based on marine products exhibited EAE (Figs. 2-3). On the other hand, among those who inhabited the inland areas of Tierra del Fuego and whose diet was primarily based on terrestrial resources, the prevalence was 1.9% (one female out of 53 crania had EAE). The prevalence difference between marine and terrestrial Fuegians was statistically not significant ($\chi2 = 2.6$; $p>0.05$) and the Chi square with Yates correction also supported this finding (1.47; p: 0.22).

Table 3. Sex distribution according to the two main areas.

	M	**F**	**Total**
Marine Fuegian	25	30	55
Terrestrial Fuegian	31	22	53
Total	56	52	108

M=Males, F= Females

Discussion

According to Kennedy (1986) the prevalence expected for EAE in an area below the 45° S latitude should be very low (<5%) compared with those of subtropical latitudes. Our results suggest that the prevalence of EAE in the Amerindians of Tierra del Fuego was very similar to the expected for the subpolar latitudes, in which they lived, and hence support Kennedy's hypothesis.

Secondly, in relation to the cold-water hypothesis, it can only be suggested that EAE may be produced by full body immersion in the cold waters that surround the island. This is supported by the ethnographical reports and our results. However, this is not supported statistically as there was no statistical difference in the

prevalence of EAE between the terrestrial and marine Fuegians. A similar thing can be said about the analysis of EAE according to sex. Although the female to male ratio of EAE was not statistically significant, the ethnographical data and our results support the evidence that women were mainly in charge of harvesting and gathering molluscs and other seafood. For instance, according to Gusinde (1961), the Yamana women provided a great contribution to the economy of the family and supplemented her husband's hunting activities by fishing and gathering shellfish. For this purpose, they used fishing lines and rowed canoes, occasionally diving down to the sea bottom to collect mussels and other marine animals. "She is not afraid of the cold water. She is used to it, because at all times of the year she must fasten her canoe a considerable distance from the beach and must swim back and forth" (Gusinde, 1961:260). Chapman (1986) has also emphasized that the Yamana and Alacaluf women rowed the canoes around the shores of the inlets and swam underneath the water to gather king crabs and other seafood whereas men were in charge of the large scale hunting of sea lions, guanacos and whales. According to Gusinde (1951) the young Yamana and Alacaluf women learnt to swim from a young age and it was rare that men could swim. On the other hand, despite the fact that their terrestrial counterparts such as the Selk'nam and Haush women were involved in fishing activities and collecting small marine animals during the low tide, there is no ethnographical evidence suggesting that they swam or dived. This fits with the low prevalence of EAE indicated by our results.

Contrary to previous studies where males have shown a higher prevalence of EAE compared to their females counterparts (Roche, 1964; Gregg and Bass, 1970; Velasco-Vazquez et al., 2000), probably as a consequence of division of labour between the sexes (Frayer, 1988; Standen et al., 1997), our data indicated the opposite. The fact that the women were in charge of practising the fishing activities, and swimming in cold waters could have a physiological explanation. Clinical studies have suggested that there is a gender-related difference in tolerance to cold-water immersion. For instance, Hong and Rahn (1976) and Graham (1988) have found that sexual differences in tolerance to cold-water exposure can be due to dimorphic thermoregulatory constituencies between the sexes. Differences in adipose tissue distribution, body mass and body surface area would make women less thermally sensitive to cold water and better suited than their male counterparts to this kind of activity.

Furthermore, most clinicians agree that it is difficult to quantify the necessary exposure to cold water to develop EAE as it depends on many variables. For instance, common related factors are the length and frequency of water exposure, such as hours spent practising aquatic sports and seasonality, as well as whether it is an 'above water sport' such as sailing or surfing or an 'underwater sport' like swimming or diving.

Age at death may have had an impact on the cases of EAE found. However, five out of six cases presenting EAE were middle adults, thus not evidencing any particular trend to manifest EAE at older ages.

The frequency with which the marine Fuegians swam in the cold water to exploit their resources cannot be precisely known. However, we can be fairly confident that they carried out such activity on a regular basis if it was a vital part of their daily survival. According to Gusinde (1961) hunting and gathering the smaller animals such as mussels and crabs constituted the chief part of the economic activity of these people. The effect of both high winds and low temperatures should not be dismissed as an influential contributory phenomenon.

Finally, as the ethnographical accounts emphasised, Selk'nams and Haush relied almost entirely on a terrestrial subsistence, therefore it is not surprising to have found only one example of EAE among them. However, according to Chapman (1986:36) the terrestrial Fuegians made use of the seafood and fish available during winter when the guanaco was lean. The exposure to cold water to compensate their diet during the cold season with marine resources could possibly explain how they developed the condition.

Conclusion

With this example it has been proved that despite the hostile and harsh cold environment of Tierra del Fuego, in particular the cold marine waters that surround the island, EAE was present below the 45° S latitude and in the southernmost land ever inhabited by man. In accordance with Kennedy's latitudinal hypothesis, the prevalence of EAE in Tierra del Fuego was very similar to the expected for sub-polar latitudes. However, as a first step for the study of EAE in populations from Tierra del Fuego, further investigations and a larger sample of marine and terrestrial Fuegians are necessary to arrive at a more definite conclusion regarding the cold water aetiology as an activity-induced pathology.

Acknowledgements

One of the authors, Miss P. Ponce would like to express her sincere appreciation to her grant sponsorship, the Durham Doctoral Fellowship Award that made this research possible.

The authors would like to express their gratitude to Mr. Diego Gobbo from the Museo of La Plata in Buenos Aires, who generously provided his help with the preparation of the map of Tierra del Fuego.

Many thanks to Mr. Robert Kruszynski from the Palaeontology department at the Natural History Museum, London, who facilitated our access to the skeletal material from Tierra del Fuego.

Literature cited

Altuna Mariezkurrena, X., Gómez Suárez, J., Luqui Albisua, I., Vea Orte, J. and Algaba Guimerá, J. 2004. "Prevalencia de exóstosis entre surfistas de la costa guipuzcoana". *Acta Otorrinolaringológica Española* 55: 364-368.

Arnay-de-la Rosa, M., Velasco-Vazquez, J., Gonzalez-Reimers, E. and Santolaria-Fernandez, F. 2001. "Auricular exostoses among the prehistoric population of different islands of the Canary archipelago". *Annals of Otology, Rhinology and Laryngology* 110: 1080-1083.

Berry, A., and Berry, B. 1967. "Epigenetic variation in the human cranium". *Journal of Anatomy* 101:361-379.

Borrero, L., Guichón, R., Tykot, R., Kelly, J., Prieto, A. and Cardenas, P. 2001. "Dieta a partir de isótopos estables en restos óseos humanos". *Anales del Instituto de la Patagonia. Serie Ciencias Humanas* 29: 119-127.

Brothwell, D. 1981. *Digging up bones: the excavation, treatment and study of human skeletal remains.* 3rd ed. Ithaca: Cornell University Press.

Buikstra, J. and Ubelaker, D. 1994. *Standards for data collection from human skeletal remains.* Fayetteville, AK: Arkansas. Archaeological Survey, Research Series No 44.

Chapman, A. 1986. *Los Selk'nam. La vida de los Onas.* Emecé ed. Argentina.

Deleyiannis, F, Cockcroft, B and Pinczower E. 1996. Exostoses of the external auditory canal in Oregon surfers. *American Journal of Otolaryngology* 17:303-307.

DiBartolomeo, J. 1979. "Exostoses of the external auditory canal". *Annals of Otology, Rhinology and Laryngology* Suppl. 88: 1-17.

Fowler, E. and Osmon, P. 1942. "New bone growth due to cold water in the ears". *Archives of Otolaryngology Head and Neck Surgery* 36: 455-466.

Frayer, D. 1988. "Auditory exostoses and evidence for fishing at Vlasac". *Current Anthropology* 29: 346-349.

García-Moro, C., Hernández, M. and Lalueza, C. 1997. "Estimation of the optimum density of the Selk'nam from Tierra del Fuego: inferences about human dynamics in extreme environments". *American Journal of Human Biology* 9: 699-708.

González-José, R., García-Moro, C., Dahinten, S. and Hernández, M. 2002. "Origin of Fuegian-Patagonians: an approach to population history and structure using R matrix and matrix permutation methods" *American Journal of Human Biology* 14: 308-320.

González-José, R. 2003. *El poblamiento de la Patagonia. Análisis de la variación craniofacial en el contexto del poblamiento Americano.* Ph.D. Dissertation. Universitat de Barcelona.

Graham, H. 1979. "Osteomatas and exostoses of the external auditory canal". *Annals of Otology, Rhinology and Laryngology* 88: 566-572.

Graham, T. 1988. "Thermal, metabolic, and cardiovascular changes in men and women during cold stress". *Medicine and Science in Sports and Exercise* Suppl 20: 185-192.

Gregg, J. and Bass, W. 1970. "Exostoses in the external auditory canals". *Annals of Otology, Rhinology and Laryngology* 70: 834-839.

Gusinde, M. 1937. *Die Feuerland Indianer.* Vienna: Verlag St. Gabriel.

Gusinde, M. 1951. *Hombres primitivos en la Tierra del Fuego: De investigador a compañero de tribu.* Escuela de Estudios Hispanoamericanos. Sevilla.

Gusinde, M. 1961. *The Yamana. The life and thought of the water nomads of Cape Horn.* New Haven: Human relations area files.

Gusinde, M. 1979. *Expedición a Tierra del Fuego.* Santiago de Chile: Editorial Universitaria.

Hanihara, T., Ishida, H. and Dodo, Y. 2003. "Characterization of biological diversity through analysis of discrete cranial traits". *American Journal of Physical Anthropology* 121: 241-251.

Hauser, G. and De Stefano, G. 1989. *Epigenetic variants of the human skull.* Stuttgart: Schweizerbart.

Hong, S. and Rahn, H. 1976. "The diving woman of Korea and Japan". In: Vander A, (ed.) *Human physiology and the environment in health and disease: readings from American Scientist.* San Francisco: W.H. Freeman. 92-102.

Hutchinson, D., Denise, C., Daniel, H. and Kalmus, G. 1997. "A re-evaluation of the cold water etiology of external auditory exostoses". *American Journal of Physical Anthropology* 103: 417-422.

Ikeda, I. 1998. "Does cold water truly promote diver's ear?" *Undersea and Hyperbaric Medicine* 25: 59-62.

Karegeannes, J. 1995. "Incidence of bony outgrowths of the external ear canal in U.S. Navy divers". *Undersea and Hyperbaric Medicine* 22: 301-306.

Kennedy, G. 1986. "The relationship between auditory exostoses and cold water: a latitudinal analysis". *American Journal of Physical Anthropology* 71: 401-415.

Kroon, D., Lawson, L., Derkay, C., Hoffmann, K. and McCook, J. 2002. "Surfer's ear: external auditory exostoses are more prevalent in cold water surfers". *Otolaryngology Head and Neck Surgery* 126: 499-504.

Lalueza, C., Pérez-Pérez, A., Prats, E., Cornudella, L. and Turbón, D. 1997. "Lack of founding Amerindian mitochondrial DNA lineages in extinct aborigines from Tierra del Fuego-Patagonia. *Human Molecular Genetics* 6: 41-46

Manzi, G., Sperduti, A. and Passarello, P. 1991. "Behaviour-induced auditory exostoses in imperial Roman society: evidence from Coeval urban and rural communities". *American Journal of Physical Anthropology* 85: 253-260.

Massone, M. and Prieto, A. 2005. "Ballenas y delfines en el mundo Selk'nam. Una aproximación etnográfica". *Magallania* 33: 25-35.

Orquera, L. and Piana, E. 1999. *La vida material y social de los Yámanas.* Buenos Aires: Eudeba.

Ossenberg, N. 1976. "Within and between race distances in population studies based on discrete traits of human skull". *American Journal of Physical Anthropology* 45: 701-716.

Perizonius, W. 1979. "Non-metric cranial traits: sex difference and age dependence". *Journal of Human Evolution* 8: 679-684.

Roche, A. 1964. "Aural exostoses in Australian aboriginal skulls". *Annals of Otology, Rhinology and Laryngology* 73: 82-91.

Seftel, D. 1977. "Ear canal hyperostosis-surfer's ear. An improved surgical technique". *Archives of Otolaryngology Head and Neck Surgery* 103: 58.

Standen, V., Arriaza, B. and Santoro, C. 1997. "External auditory exostosis in prehistoric Chilean populations: a test of the cold water hypothesis". *American Journal of Physical Anthropology* 103: 119-129.

Timofeev, I., Notkina, N. and Smith, I. 2004. "Exostoses of the external auditory canal: a long-term follow-up study of surgical treatment". *Clinical Otolaryngology* 29: 588-594.

Velasco-Vazquez, J., Betancor-Rodríguez, A., Arnay-de-la Rosa, M. and Gonzalez-Reimers, E. 2000. "Auricular exostoses in the prehistoric population of Gran Canaria". *American Journal of Physical Anthropology* 112:49-55.

Yesner, D., Figuerero Torres, M., Guichón, R. and Borrero, L. 2003. "Stable isotope analysis of human bone and ethnohistoric subsistence patterns in Tierra del Fuego". *Journal of Anthropological Archaeology* 22: 279-291.

West Butts Street cemetery, Poole: a small 18th century Baptist community

Jacqueline I. McKinley

Wessex Archaeology, Portway House, Old Sarum Park,
Salisbury, Wiltshire, SP4 6EB
e-mail address for correspondence: j.mckinley@wessexarch.co.uk

Abstract

In 1735, a small community of Baptists – comprising 15 named individuals - living in the thriving Dorset port of Poole, joined together to organise the construction of a meeting house, the enclosed area around which functioned as their burial ground. On the death of their one and only minister c. 53 years later the community dwindled and faltered, and the chapel was demolished. The small number of remaining Baptists worshiped at another Nonconformist meeting house in the town prior to forming their own community in 1804. Their new church and burial ground were not established until 1815 and in the meantime they continued to use the West Butts Street cemetery for disposal of their dead.

Full excavation of the West Butts cemetery in 2003 recovered the remains of 100 individuals, representing a discrete community of early Nonconformists. Despite extensive documentary research, providing a wealth of information about 18th century Poole, its population and economic status, frustratingly little has emerged about the members of this early Baptist community or the life of the chapel; demonstrating one of the difficulties of dealing with early Nonconformist groups. It has, however, been possible to form an impression of the world in which the members of the congregation lived and worshipped, and at least some of the factors which would have influenced their lives. This paper focuses on several interesting features of the demographic make-up of the cemetery population, specifically the imbalance between the sexes and the number of infants.

Keywords: 18th century, Baptists, maritime trade

Introduction

This paper will focus on two specific aspects of the demographic data recovered from the cemetery at West Butts Street, Poole, the population of which represents a discrete community of 18th century Nonconformists. The aim is to demonstrate how a combination of osteological, archaeological and historical data can inform each other to illustrate the social organisation, position and lifestyle of those who chose to distinguish themselves from their contemporaries in terms of their religious practice. The paper will give some impression of the range of documentary sources available for this period relating to a population within a provincial town, particularly compared with the larger cities where most similar work has hitherto been undertaken (e.g. Molleson and Cox, 1993; Brickley and Miles, 1999; Brickley and Buteux, 2006). It should also highlight the difficulties in tracing detailed information about some Nonconformist groups, particularly the Baptists who – somewhat frustratingly – often failed to 'conform' in terms of keeping records.

18th century Poole

The port of Poole is situated on the Dorset coast, c. 25 km south-west of Southampton (Fig. 1). Its excellent location, on an alluvial peninsula (almost an island until the later 19th century) at the head of a large natural harbour, means that it has been exploited as a port from at least the 12th century, being included in a list of the principal ports of England in the 13th century (Sydenham,

1839:351; Smith, 1948; 1951; Penn, 1980:82; Legg, 2005:17).

Although already an important harbour, Poole increased considerably in size and prosperity throughout the 18th century, largely, though not exclusively, on account of trade with Newfoundland. In 1787 the port was ranked 11th of the 73 English and Welsh ports. Between 1787 and 1792 it averaged 79 vessels per year to the Newfoundland fishery and acted as the chief supplier of goods to the colonists

> "… nets, cordage, sail-cloth, and all sorts of wearing apparel, with a variety of other commodities…Their returns are in cod and salmon sent to foreign markets, oil, seal-skins, furs, and lately cran-berries are become an article for home consumption …" (Barfoot and Wilkes, 1798:239; Davies, 1994).

There was also a steady trade with South Carolina and the Leeward Islands with 41 vessels clearing for voyages in 1720-1 and 84 in 1751-2 (ibid.). In the middle years of the century merchants were importing up to 47,000 gallons of wine per year as return cargo from the Mediterranean; though many ships in the Mediterranean traded there for years without returning home (ibid.). Following the settlement in 1763 at the end of the wars with France, Poole shipping expanded dramatically and by 1789 over 200 vessels were engaged in foreign trade with a further 966 inward and outward coastal cargoes. Fishing was also an important commercial enterprise both

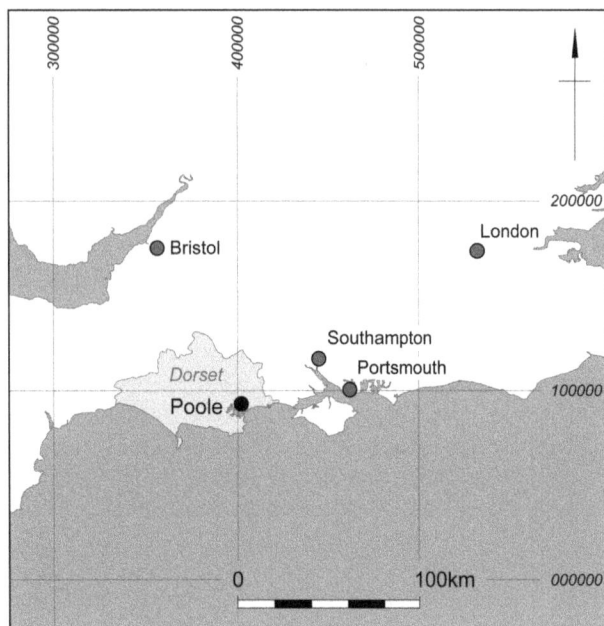

Figure 1. Location map of Poole.

for home consumption and export, particularly oysters. Other fish were "...caught in great pleanty, and the harbour plaice are most excellent. Herrings have been caught in such pleanty as to be sold for a penny a dozen, and continue on our coast for three months" (Barfoot and Wilkes, 1798: 241).

A vast network of mercantile trading and associated manufacture developed in response to the maritime trade, the effects of which spread to the surrounding region, and the inhabitants of Poole were regarded to be of "... great opulence and respectability" (Davies, 1994). The relatively small size of many of the vessels and consequent small scale of the shares in shipping encouraged the small investor, and several of Poole's minor tradespeople were able to benefit directly from the maritime trade by purchasing part-shares in ships (*ibid.*). Most of the town's inhabitants were engaged in some sort of trade or manufacturing, the majority linked with the maritime enterprises - rope makers, shipwrights, blacksmiths, carpenters, coopers, sail makers and victuallers as well as the more obvious sailors – the latter of which, by the end of the 18th century, probably comprised 21% of the population. The town's prosperity is well illustrated by the fine 18th century public buildings as well as a considerable number of grand private dwellings which can still be seen (Fig. 2).

Throughout most of its history the harbour - the Great and Little Quays - was situated on the south side of the peninsula, with the main part of the town clustered behind it (Fig. 3). West Butts Street lay on the north-west margins of the town, on the late-medieval/early post-medieval reclaimed foreshore overlooking Longfleet Bay and the Backwater channel.

The West Butts Street Baptists

Poole was a royal peculiar, exempt from the usual Episcopal supervision and geographically isolated from the Bishop's seat in Bristol (Densham and Ogle, 1899: 181). Its inhabitants were largely engaged in prosperous trade, and exposed to social, political and religious influences from continental Europe and the New World. This independence of the town and its people gave the population a degree of freedom from external control to follow their Nonconformist inclinations, and Nonconformity flourished in Poole from the mid-17th century onwards.

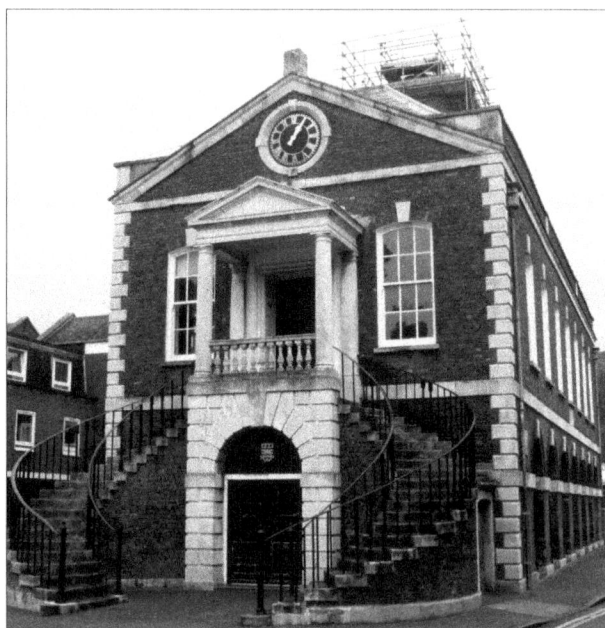

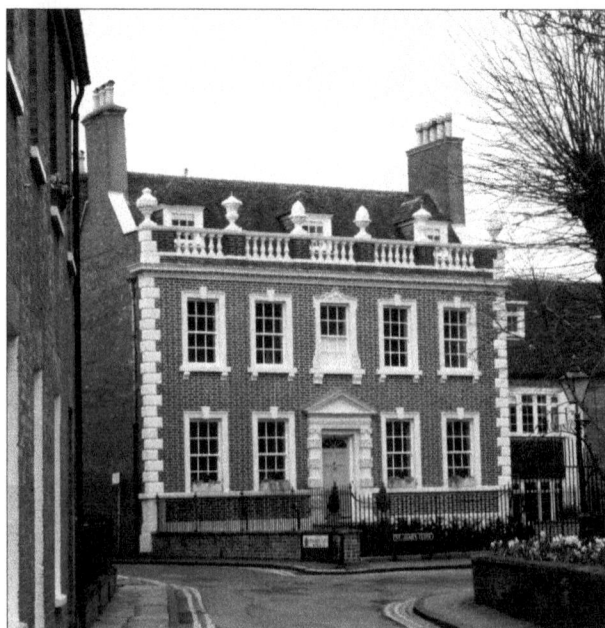

Figure 2. 18th century buildings in Poole: the guildhall and one of the several private mansion houses.

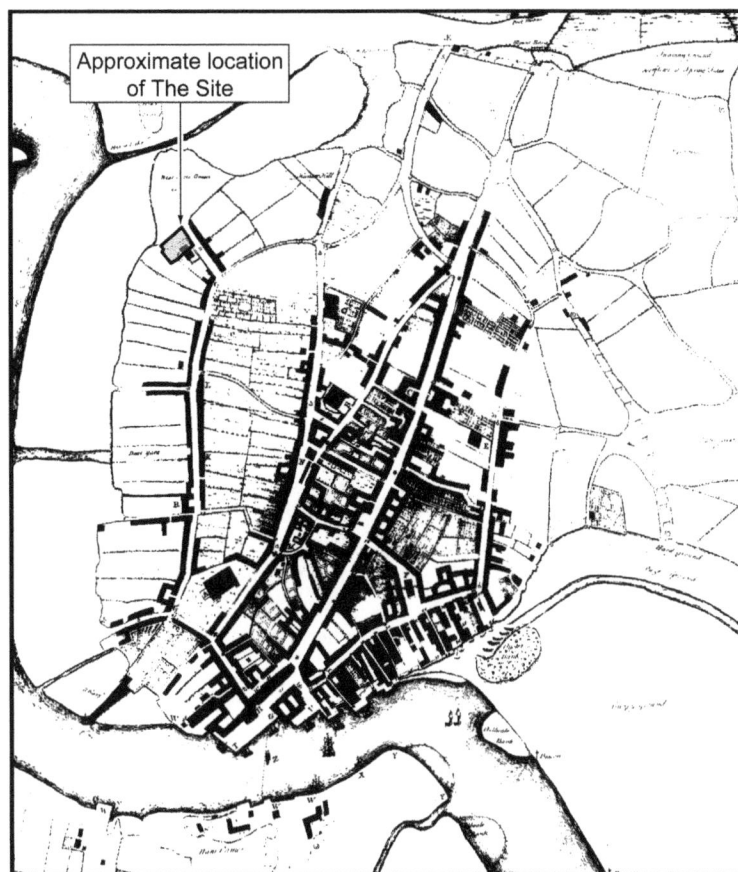

Figure 3. Thompson's 1751 map of Poole showing the West Butts Street chapel and burial Ground (courtesy Poole Museum).

The rector of St. James Parish Church in 1642 is recorded to have had "strong Presbyterian sympathies" (Densham and Ogle, 1899:181). When the 1661 Corporation Act (requiring those wishing to hold municipal office to produce evidence that they took communion at their parish church) came into effect the mayor, water bailiff, recorder and 17 other of the town's municipal office holders were ejected since "Many of them were well-known Nonconformists" (*ibid*.:183). John Wesley, grandfather of the founders of Methodism, was amongst the many Dorset ministers who lost their livings following the 1662 Act of Uniformity (requiring all ministers to publicly assent to the exclusive use of the Book of Common Prayer), and subsequently became a regular preacher in Poole (Densham and Ogle, 1899:184-5). Poole's first purpose-built Dissenting place of worship was licensed in 1705-6 (Hutchins, 1861:60) and in 1735, Bishop Secker's diocesan survey of Dorset recorded that there was a majority of 'Dissenters' in the parish of St. James (Bettey, 1973:74).

Relatively little is known about the early Baptist movement in Poole. It is probable that a private house "…licensed for an assembly for religious worship…" in 1707 was used for Baptist meetings (Sydenham, 1839: 346) and many Baptists used the town's other Nonconformist meeting house (see above; Short, 1927: 57); such inter-communion obviously being considered quite acceptable to both parties in the absence of a more

suitable alternative. It is possible that there was more than one group of Baptists in Poole in the early 18th century, though the size of any one group may have been very small. West Butts Street was registered as a Baptist place of worship on 6th November 1735 (RG31/8 National Archives, Kew). Although the original covenant, a photocopy of which survives (Fig. 4), mentions that the 15 founding members formerly belonged to "… severall Congregations at great distance now living in & about the Town & County of Poole …", the new congregation is also likely to have included several of the town's existing inhabitants.

The West Butts Street congregation only ever had one Minster – Mr. Bird – and as his health failed in the 1770s the congregation dwindled, and following his death in 1788 the chapel was demolished. It was originally thought that the burial ground ceased to be used at the same time, but documentary evidence and the recovery during the excavations of a partially legible coffin plate dated 1813/?8 showed this was not the case (Fig. 5). A new Baptist congregation, apparently incorporating some of the former West Butts Street Baptists who had been worshipping at one of the town's other Nonconformist Churches, was established in 1804 (Johnson and McKinley, forthcoming). It appears that the West Butts cemetery had been and continued to be used by the Baptists following the closure of the chapel in 1789 up until the establishment of a new burial ground attached to the Hill Street Church constructed in 1815. The burial ground is, therefore, likely to have been used over about an 80 year period and to have served two Baptist - albeit tenuously connected - congregations.

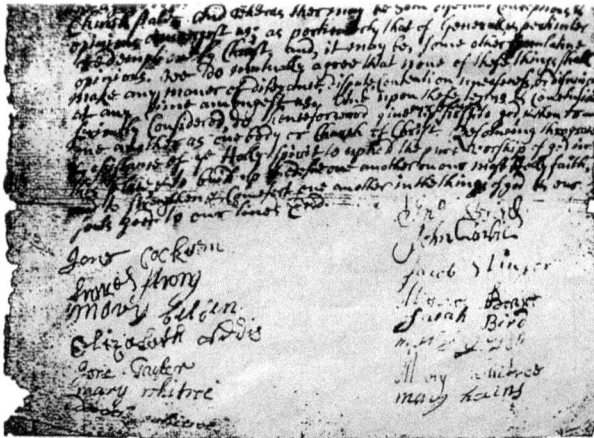

Figure 4. Lower portion of the 1735 West Butts Street Baptist covenant showing the 15 signatures (courtesy Hill Street Baptists).

Excavations

Following its final closure in 1854, as part of the national-wide initiative to close all town-centre burial grounds for health reasons, the cemetery walls continued to be maintained and the area respected, remaining under the ownership of the Hill Street Baptists until at least the early part of the 20th century (Johnson and McKinley, forthcoming; Fig. 6). Some use had been made of the area for storage purposes but little or no intrusive disturbance had occurred other than on the south-east and possibly the northern margins in the middle to latter part of last century (*ibid.*). Following the purchase of the land by the Royal National Lifeboat Institute (RNLI) in the 1970s and subsequent demolition of the surrounding buildings, the area had been used as a car park.

Consequently, when Wessex Archaeology came to undertake the excavations of the site in 2003 in advance of the construction of the new Lifeboat Support Centre (part of the RNLI headquarters in Poole), most, if not all of the cemetery is known to have survived intact. The *in situ* remains of 83 burials were recovered, with a MNI 100 for the assemblage as a whole. Figure 7 shows the predominant (92.6%) southwest-northeast alignment of the burials, an orientation which appears to have been influenced by the position of West Butts Street to which most of the graves were set at right-angles. One grave (222; Fig. 7) on a similar alignment to the rest contained the remains of a burial made northeast-southwest; possibly the result of the coffin having accidentally been placed the wrong way round in the grave. Four graves were cut at right-angles to the majority, on the same alignment as West Butts Street; three of the burials had been made southeast-northwest (graves 165, 173, 247 Fig. 7) and one northwest-southeast (grave 121). Although the accepted traditional form for Christian

burial is west-east, there are rare examples of deviations from this norm even in medieval cemeteries (Gilchrist and Sloane, 2005:152-3) and several graves in some other 18th-19th century Nonconformist cemeteries show similar deviations to those at West Butts (Bashford and Pollard, 1998:159).

Other than a copy of the original West Butts covenant very little other direct documentary evidence survives for the community. There are no burial records for the cemetery. It has not been possible to trace any of the individuals named in the covenant from the Parish Records or wills, and Pastor Bird does not feature amongst the contemporary lists of Baptist ministers for Dorset (Johnson and McKinley, forthcoming). This lack of records, particularly from early Baptist communities, is not particularly unusual and in part reflects the nature of Baptist churches. Unlike most other Nonconformist groups each Baptist church forms a separate, self-governing body and there is no central headquarters where systemised records of ministers and local churches are kept (Breed, 1995:1-3). Individual churches may choose whether to join organisations such as area assemblies or not. An extant church may keep its own records or may have deposited them elsewhere. Where churches/congregations no longer exist records may be found at County Records Offices, the Angus Library (Baptist Archive, Regents Park College, Oxford) or may remain in private hands. Unfortunately, for the purpose of this research, the West Butts congregation seems to have elected to be independent. Consequently, despite the alluring existence of references to its date of establishment and those who formed the initial core of its congregation, any further information pertaining to the church or records associated with or alluding to it, either never existed or have not survived.

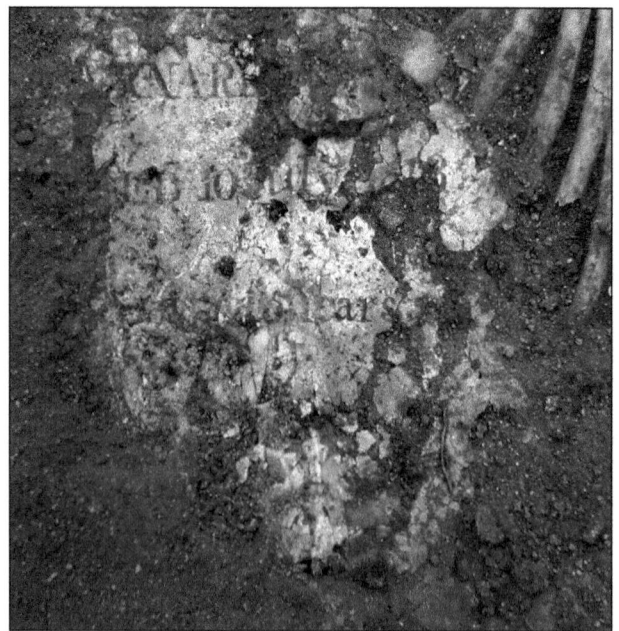

Figure 5. Partly legible breast plate from grave 379.

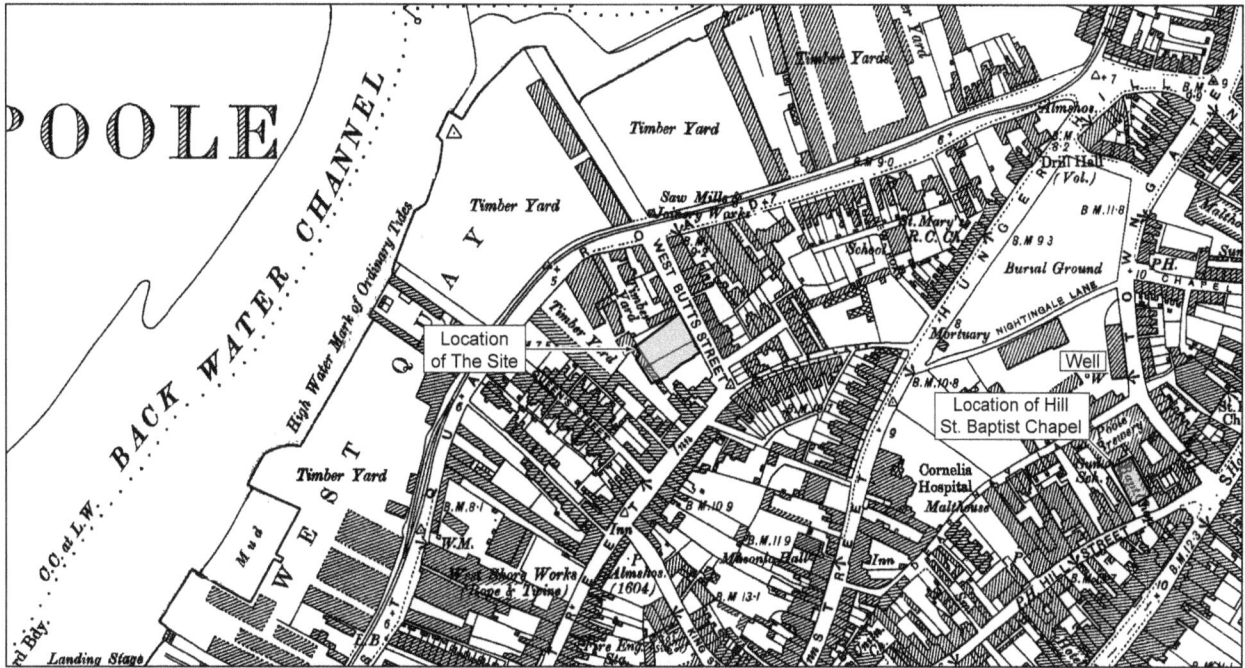

Figure 6. Second edition Ordnance Survey (1902) showing location of burial ground.

Biographical data recovered from the coffins was similarly sparse. Most were simple with limited information about the deceased – initials, age at death, date of death – shown in upholstery studs (or in two cases sheet iron letters) inserted into the coffin lid, which had invariably become illegible as the coffin collapsed (Fig. 8). Breast plates were recovered from four graves but only one was partly legible (Fig. 5). Little close-dating evidence survived in any of the graves. The coffin furniture (grips, grip plates, copper alloy studs, iron sheet letters and breast plates) generally appear to be of local (Poole) manufacture, of a type in common use in the provinces, and with a lengthy post-medieval currency (Mepham and Every, forthcoming). The technique of using upholstery pins to spell out biographical details was most common before 1730, but its use clearly continued throughout the 18th century in provincial areas where coffins are likely to have been built by local carpenters using old techniques (*ibid.*). Fully legible dates of death survived in only two cases – grave 261 (1772) and grave 379 (1813/?8) – with partial dates in three others; all were 18th century. Consequently, the chronology of the cemetery is only relative and based on discrete stratigraphic relationships (McKinley and Egging, forthcoming).

Gender difference

During the course of the excavation it was noticeable that many of the skeletons were those of females; an impression that was confirmed during osteological analysis when it was found that there was a substantially higher ratio of females (61%) to males (36%) amongst the adults (Table 1). The figures appear in stark contrast to most other contemporaneous cemeteries which show a much closer similarity between the sexes (Table 2). It may be significant that a similar disparity (though the

overall numbers are small) was seen in the only other Baptist cemetery in the sample also located within a port. A combination of factors are likely to be reflected in the figures from West Butts relating both to the creed of the community and its maritime economy.

Females appear to have played an important role –if non-ministerial and excluded from the official 'running' of the chapel - within early Nonconformist communities in which they commonly considerably out-numbered men. Of the 15 signatories to the 1735 West Butts covenant drawn-up on the congregation's formation (Fig. 4), 11 were female and only four male (an almost 3:1 ratio); only one couple featured, the minister and his wife - John and Sarah Bird. Similar discrepancies can be observed in a number of early Baptist communities in west Wiltshire (the adjacent county to the north of Dorset; Fig. 1) where in small groups of founder members the women often outnumbered the men. For example, Penknap was founded in 1810 with 30 people (17 females, 13 males); in 1812, 49 members (32 females, 17 males) of the Back Street Church in Trowbridge withdrew, 41 of them (27 females, 14 males) forming a new church the following year (Doel, 1890). Elsewhere numbers were more even, e.g. Beckington founded in 1786 with 16 (eight females and eight males) and Chapmanslade in 1788 with nine (five females and four males; *ibid.*). On a few occasions, of course, the men did outnumber the women e.g. at Hilperton 1806 with ten (three females, seven males; *ibid.*).

This discrepancy in numbers of females to males may, in part, have been a matter of inclination, females being more drawn to the Nonconformist faiths; however, until the repeal of the 1661 Corporations Act in the 19th century, with its political, social and economic consequences for males if they declared their membership

113

Table 1. Summary of age and sex distributions.

Immature							
	Unsexed	Female			Male			Total
		??	?	total	??	?	total	
foetus <full term	2							2
neonate 0-6 mth.	2							2
infant 0.5-5 yr.	17							17
juvenile 5-12 yr.	4							4
subadult 13-18 yr.	1			1	1		1	3
Totals				1	1		1	28
Adult								
	Unsexed	Female			Male			Total
		??	?	total	??	?	total	
>18 yr.	1							1
> 25 yr.	1							1
c. 18-25 yr.				2				2
c. 18-45 yr.			1	1				1
c. 25-40 yr.				1		1	1	2
c. 30-45 yr.		1		8		1	4	12
c. 30-55 yr.		1		5		1	7	12
c. 40-55 yr.			1	7			2	9
c. 40-60 yr.		1	1	9	1	1	6	15
>45 yr.						2	3	3
c. 50-70 yr.			1	4	1		2	6
> 50 yr.		1	1	7	1		1	9
Totals	2	3	5	**44**	5	4	**26**	**72**

of a Nonconformist congregation and refused communion with the Church of England, it may have been a matter of necessity. The males could not officially 'join' if they aspired to any public office, but their wives, widows and daughters might do so.

This may have been exacerbated in the 17th and first half of the 18th century by the firmly rooted General Baptist[1] tradition of endogamy (i.e. marriage within the 'tribe').

'... for decades frustrated sisters within these churches probably kept the topic [of endogamy] alive and urgent ... During the next twenty-five years [following renewed debates in 1719] the scene gradually changed but not without considerable personal distress and an unnecessary depletion of their [Baptist] membership ...' (Brown, 1986:19-20).

It is probable that, at least in the early days of the West Butts congregation, this dictat was still enforced and that some of the 11 female signatories were and remained

spinsters, in common with other female members of the congregation. Although not necessarily reflective of the Baptist congregation, a review of Prerogative Court of Canterbury (PCC) wills for Poole between 1750 and 1800 shows approximately 6% to be those of spinsters (National Archive Document). A further consequence of this, of course, would be fewer new 'members' being born into the congregation (see below).

In the period covered by the cemetery, sea-trade - both coastal and particularly international - was expanding in Poole (see above). Sailors could be away for months or often years at a time (at least two ships are recorded as being away 4-6 years; Davies, 1994). Documentary evidence for the potential size of the population of Poole in the 18th century suggests slightly variable figures depending on the source and - possibly more pertinent - the apparent inclusion or exclusion of a large transitory population of seamen. Data from 1766 gives a figure of "...near 7000 inhabitants..." stipulating the figure is for "...when the Newfoundland ships came home ..." (Hutchins, 1803:450). The *Universal Directory* for 1798 (Barfoot and Wilkes) states that around 1500 men were employed in shipping but only 140 of the 230 ships referenced as belonging to the port were engaged in foreign trade - the rest being used in coastal trade and fishing - which substantially reduces the potential number of long-term absentee citizens to a rough estimate of 900-1000. In an 1801 census of the town, the gender divide within the population gives a slightly higher

---

[1] In the first two centuries of their history the English Baptist movement had two distinct denominations divided by theology and, to a lesser extent, practice. The General Baptists theology was Arminian (after Jacobus Arminius, 1610, who rejected the Calvinistic doctrine of predestination; Cross and Livingstone, 1997:107) and their polity was allied with the Presbyterians (*ibid.* 660). Particular Baptist theology was essentially Calvinistic (with its characteristic emphasis on predestination, though the doctrine was not central to the system; *ibid.* 268). Their polity was similar to that of the Independents but with an emphasis on 'associations' of local Churches.

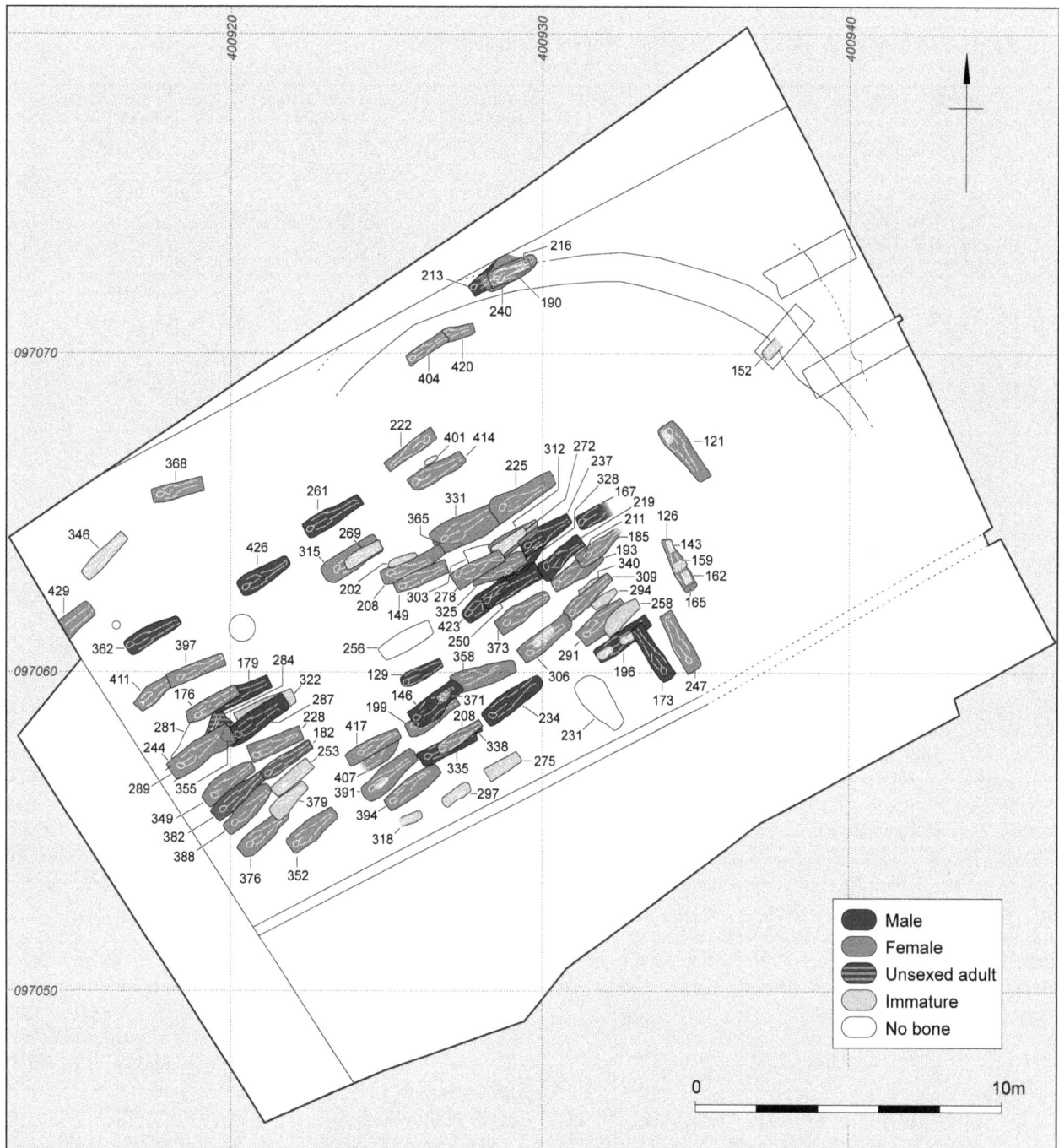

Figure 7. Cemetery plan showing grave and burial orientations, and distribution by sex and age groups.

proportion of females (55%) to males (45%). However, the overall population figures of close to 5000 viewed in conjunction with figure of *c.* 7000 given by Hutchin's for 1766 (see above), suggests the former may have been exclusive of many of those individuals absent on a long-term voyages (Sydenham, 1839: 450; N.B. the returns included only those individuals in occupation of the property on the night of the census). If this was the case and the potential number of such individuals to be included (see above), the gender divide would be slightly redressed to about 54% males and 46% females. Both sets of figures, however, illustrate the abnormal imbalance between the sexes within the West Butts population.

There is little documentary evidence for the occupation of the members of the West Butts congregation but it is likely, in this major sea-port – where up to 21% of the population were mariners (see previous paragraph) – that at least some will have been seamen, both Naval and merchant. The PCC Wills for Poole between 1750 and 1800, representative of the middle and upper end of the social strata, show approximately 17% to be those of mariners, again both Naval and merchant (National Archive Document). In addition to individuals being overcome by illness whilst away from home or death from injuries sustained during the course of their normal duties at sea, shipwrecks were common, with losses due to storms or navigational errors to both long-route traders

Table 2. Demographic data from some contemporaneous cemeteries.

Cemetery	date range	sample size	adults (>18 yr.)	immature (<18 yr.)
West Butts, Poole	1735-c.1815	100	72 (72%) F: 44 (61%), M: 26 (35%)	26 (26%)
St. Nicholas's, Sevenoaks, Kent (Boyle & Keevill, 1993)	1550-1875	192	175 (91%) F: 61 (35%), M: 55 (31%)	17 (9%)
Spitalfields, London (Molleson & Cox 1993, 23-26)	1729-1852	968	623 (64%) F: 312 (50%), M: 311 (50%)	251 (26%)
St. Brides, London (Scheuer 1998)	1740-1852	227	212 (93%) F: 103 (49%), M: 109 (51%)	15 (7%)
St. Martin's, Birmingham (Brickley 2006, table 92)	late 18th C – 19th C	505	352 (70%) F: 130 (37%), M: 180 (51%)	153 (30%)
Friends Burial Ground, Kings Lynn, Norfolk (Mahoney 2005)	late 18th C– early 19thC	34	32 (94%) F: 16 (50%), M: 15 (47%)	2 (6%)
Baptist Burial Ground, Kings Lynn, Norfolk (Boston 2005)	early-mid 19th C	17	15 (88%) F: 9 (60%), M: 7 (40%)	2 (12%)
Cross Bones, Southwark, London (Brickley and Miles 1999, table 5)	mid 19th C	148	*45 (30%) F: 20 (44%), M: 21 (47%)	*103 (70%)

M: Male, F: Female. * slight overlap in immature/adult age ranges

and (predominantly) those working the coastal waters (McKee, 1974:236). There was also the threat of French privateers in the Channel (the country was at war with France in the 1740s and 1750s, the Revolutionary and Napoleonic wars stretching over 25 years at the end of the period of reference) and Barbary corsairs in the Mediterranean (Davies, 1994); the crews of captured vessels may be imprisoned, impressed or killed. All such dangers at sea undoubtedly led to the loss of life which would not be marked by a grave on land, and most, if not all, such losses would be of males. Consequently, even if the West Butts congregation did include proportionate numbers of males to females, some, if not many of the former may not have been afforded a burial within the cemetery.

Family size

Bills of Mortality for 18th century London show that over 30% of deaths occurred in the first two years of life, with approximately 40% between 0-5 years and roughly 50% before the age of 20 years (Roberts and Cox, 2003:303-4, table 6.5). Such figures are rarely reflected in the osteological demographic profiles of contemporaneous cemeteries either from London or elsewhere (Table 2); a variety of intrinsic (poor preservation/survival, shallow immature graves) and extrinsic (age-related cultural variations) factors are commonly cited to explain the discrepancies. There are, obviously, limitations in the comparisons which can be drawn between the nation's capital and a seaport on the Dorset coast; different stresses would be brought to bear on individuals living in the dense urban environment of London and those of the thriving and expanding but still comparatively small seaport with its ready access to a rural hinterland and (relatively) fresh sea-air. Living conditions and dietary stresses, particularly those experienced by the poor, will

still have taken their toll, however, as demonstrated by mortality rates from the Dorset port of Lyme Regis (approx. 68 km/45 miles to the west of Poole) for the first half of the 19th century. These indicate 40% of deaths occurring between 0-15 years and records for 1849 show close to 20% occurring in the first year (Walker, 1981). Smallpox, measles and whooping cough were amongst the commonest cause of childhood deaths (*ibid.*), representing only some amongst the universally distributed acute infections which left no marks on the bone.

The proportion of immature to adult individuals from West Butts are similar to those recorded in some other contemporaneous cemeteries (Table 1). Most of the immature individuals were less than five years old (75%; 21% of total population; Table 1), with a substantial proportion of two years or less (46% immature; 13% of total population). So, whereas the overall number of individuals may appear low, the distribution within that group appears similar to the 'normal' pattern suggested by the London Bills of Mortality and Lyme Regis data discussed above.

At West Butts we know we had the entire population (see above *Excavations*) and the apparent overall dearth of immature individuals cannot be blamed on poor preservation as even foetal remains were well preserved and represented. All except two of the *in situ* burials were coffined. Most immature individuals were buried in an individual grave; one neonate was buried in the same coffin as an adult female (grave 391), and two infants and one juvenile were interred directly above the coffin of an adult (graves 196 (infant and juvenile) and 306). Other than a cluster of three infant's graves at the south end of the site (graves 318, 297 and 275; Fig. 7) there was little distinction in terms of the location of the graves of

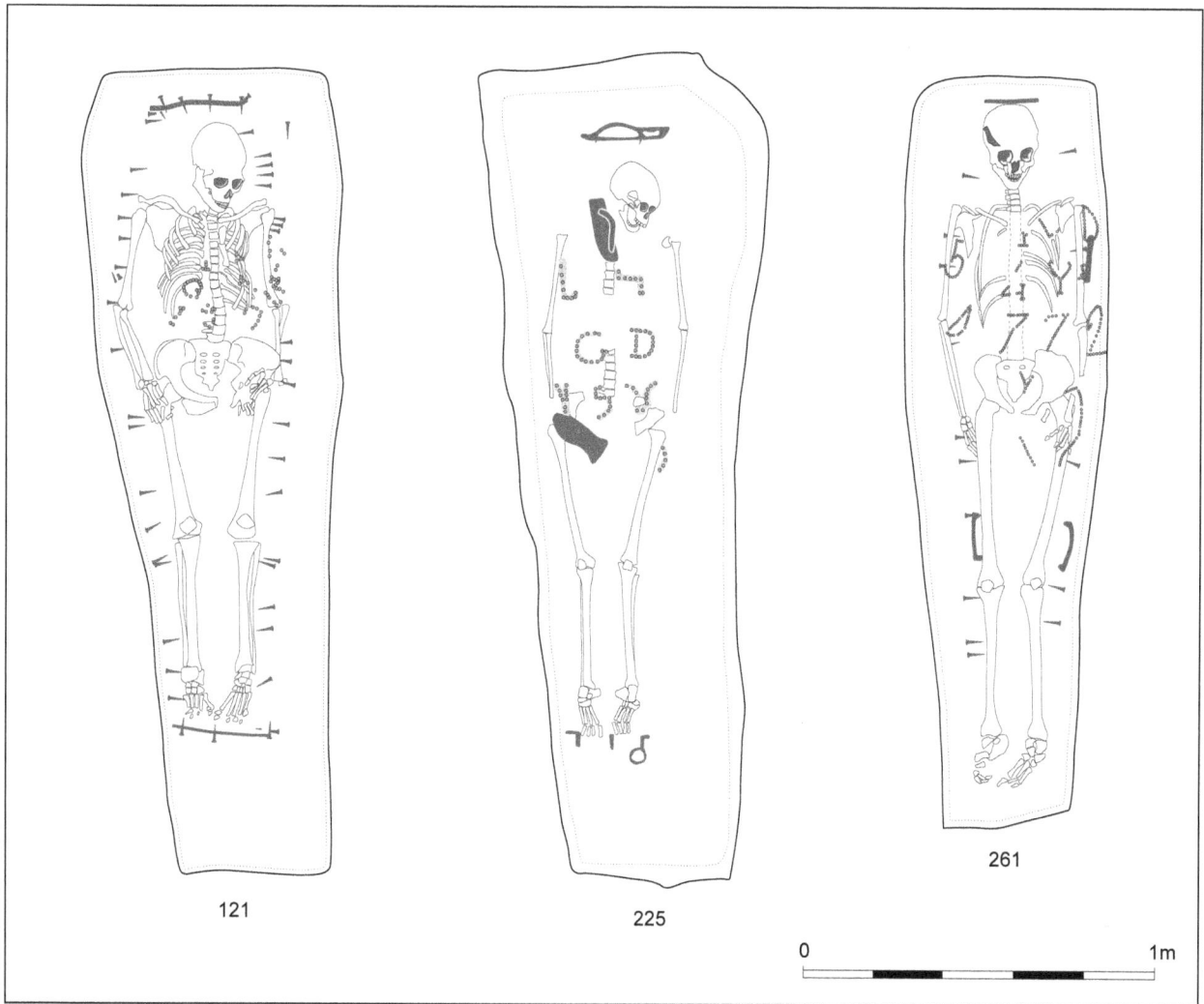

Figure 8. Selection of grave plans.

immature individuals; as with the rest of the graves the temporal distribution was largely undecernable (see above *Excavations*). It is possible that there were more young individuals amongst the disturbed and redeposited remains than is apparent within the MNI. The identified redeposited infants were sometimes represented by very little bone and it is possible that some were lost by this mechanism. Against this should be balanced the fairlysmall size of the cemetery, its known limited temporal range and the relatively low frequency of intercutting burials or other intrusions causing disturbance to the bone (no 'cemetery soil' as such). In this instance it is likely that the observed rates are close to a true reflection of the population utilising the cemetery.

The low overall numbers of immature individuals may be related to the factors reflected by imbalance between the sexes within the cemetery discussed earlier. A preponderance of females, a larger than average proportion of whom may never have married or were married to seamen who spent a substantial amount of time away from home, could both have lead to fewer and smaller families.

Entries for Poole in the *Militia Ballot Lists* (Medlycott, 1999), compiled in the second half of the 18th century, occasionally included comments with regard to a man's family. Recording was inconsistent and only 280 of the 1057 entries for Poole include any family detail; whether or not the man had a wife and how many children they had. This, presumably random, sample does, however, illustrate the probable average family size at this time (Table 3). Males with more than four children under the age of ten years were amongst those exempt ('crossed-out') from inclusion in the list, so there was potentially an inverted pressure to over- rather than under-play the size of one's family (*ibid.* 1). Large families - due to accident or choice - do not appear to have been common. The highest percentage of households appear to have included three children with a median number of two. The *Militia Ballot Lists* included males of 18-50 years and the individual's age was not recorded; consequently, it may have included a high proportion of young married men who's families had not yet reached their full number.

What would not be reflected in the figures from the *Ballot Lists*, of course, are children who had been born into the family but not survived. The period over which the cemetery was mostly in use falls before the 1837

Table 3. Number of children listed as family members in Dorset Militia Ballot Lists for late 18th century Poole.

Number of children	0	1	2	3	4	5	6	7	8
Number of 'households'	59	62	40	64	35	10	8	1	1
	21.7%	22.1%	14.3%	22.9%	12.5%	3.6%	2.9%	0.4%	0.4%

introduction of the national system of registration of births, deaths and marriages in England and Wales, and consequently the parish register for Poole St. James provides the only potential source of further information pertaining to the number of births and death in the parish. bounds of this project (the age at death was not consistently stated anyway). Overall numbers of baptisms and burials for several years during the 18th century are given by Sydenham (1839: 451) and show a steady rise between 1740 and 1800 in the number of both – baptisms 49-139, burials 30-133 - but there is no demographic detail.

Osteological indicators of childhood stress at West Butts do not give a consistent picture. Relatively low rates of dental enamel hypoplasia (prevalence rate (TPR) 23%, crude prevalence rate (CPR) 48%) suggest infants and young children were generally well nourished and not subject to repeated stress from illness, possibly benefiting from the longer period of breast-feeding within the range common for the period (Lewis, 2007 6.4; McKinley, forthcoming). Rates of *cribra orbitalia* (TPR 15.86%, CPR 15%) and rickets (CPR 10%, TPR tibia lesions 8.86%/femoral lesions 6.74%) suggest a more median position in comparison with other contemporary sites, and that at least a proportion of those burying their dead at the site suffered various vitamin deficiencies in childhood.

Concluding remarks

The West Butts cemetery population offers a discrete view of a particular section of the population of a provincial 18th century English port; these individuals were distinguished from their fellow citizens by their religious beliefs. The demographic data from the cemetery shows an intriguing discrepancy between the numbers of males and females within the population combined with an apparent low fertility rate, the two observations being potentially associated. An understanding of the form and nature of early Baptist communities, together with the location and economic status of the town of Poole, have assisted in suggesting factors which were probably of significance in producing the cemetery's demographic make-up.

The unusually high ratio of females to males is likely to have been affected by a combination of two major factors; aspects of the early Baptist creed and the congregation's location in a thriving and busy seaport. Females are recorded as commonly outnumbering males in early Nonconformist congregations, though the reasons for this discrepancy are unclear. They may simply have been more attracted to the creed or males (including close

Unfortunately, the register was transcribed in alphabetical order by the local Family History Society rather than by year and a comprehensive search would have been very time-consuming and could not be undertaken within the

relations of female members) may have been dissuaded from joining due to the attendant proscription against the holding of any public office encoded in the 1661 Corporations Act. In addition to this there may have been an unusually high number of unmarried women in the congregation due to the early Baptist practice of endogamy, the latter undoubtedly being exacerbated by the aforementioned factors. In a town with such a flourishing sea-trade and so many of its occupants (potentially 21%) working as sailors, at least some of the males within the congregation are likely to have been mariners. Shipwrecks and loss of life at sea were very common in the 18th century, for both coastal and deep-sea shipping, and it is, therefore, probable that some of the congregation's males could not be afforded burial within the West Butts cemetery. These factors would not have been mutually exclusive, but any of them could have contributed towards the observed imbalance between females and males within the cemetery.

The apparent low fertility rate could reflect the same causes as those affecting the higher numbers of females within the cemetery population. Women who remained unmarried either out of choice or as a consequence of being unable to find a suitable Baptist partner would not produce children. The families of mariner's engaged on long-term voyages to the Mediterranean and the New World would not have the potential to increase at the same rate as those of permanent residents.

The aim of this paper has been to try and demonstrate how the various forms of documentary data pertaining, however obliquely, to an individual cemetery and the osteological data may inform on one another to create an overall picture of a social group. In this instance the demographic data has been used as an example but similar informed discussion can follow on from metric and pathological data. The lessons learned from such exercises undertaken on material from the historic period may also assist the osteologist to reflect on factors which may have affected earlier, non-historic assemblages.

Acknowledgements

The archaeological excavations were commissioned by Ellis Belk Associates, on behalf of their clients the Royal National Lifeboat Institute (RNLI), who funded the project. Much of the documentary research was undertaken by Sue Johnson who is to be acknowledge for her diligence. Access to unpublished human bone reports by Ceri Boston and D. Mahoney of Oxford Archaeology is appreciated. Grateful thanks are also due to Reverend Sally Parker, Ralph Thomas and Joan Orme, of the Hill Street Baptist congregation, for access to their archive. The drawings were prepared for publication by Rob Goller.

Literature cited

Barfoot, P. and Wilkes, J. (eds.) 1798. *The Universal British Directory of Trade, Commerce and Manufacture etc.* London: Champante & Whitrow.

Bashford, L. and Pollard, T. 1998. " 'In the burying place' – the excavation of a Quaker burial ground". In: Cox, M. (ed.) *Grave Concerns. Death and Burial in England 1700-1850.* York: Council for British Archaeology Research Report 113. 154-166.

Bettey, J.H. 1973. "Bishop Secker's Diocesan Survey" *Dorset Natural History and Archaeological Society Proceedings* 95: 74-75.

Boston, C. 2005 "Human bone - Baptist inhumations" In: Brown, R. *Vancouver Centre and Clough Lane Car Park, King's Lynn, Norfolk. Post excavation Assessment and Updated Project Design.* Oxford Archaeology (unpublished).

Boyle, A. and Keevil, G. 1993. " 'To the praise of the dead, and anatomie': the analysis of post-medieval burials at St. Nicholas, Sevenoaks, Kent". In: Cox, M. (ed.) *Grave Concerns. Death and burials in England 1700-1850.* York: Council for British Archaeology Research Report 113. 85-96.

Breed, G. 1995. *My Ancestors Were Baptists.* London: Society of Genealogists.

Brickley, M. 2006: "The People: Physical Anthropology". In: Brickley, M. and Buteux, S. *St. Martin's Uncovered: Investigations in the Churchyard of St. Martin's-in-the-Bull-Ring, Birmingham, 2001.* Oxford: Oxbow. 90-151.

Brickley, M. and Miles, A. 1999 *The Cross Bones Burial Ground, Redcross Way, Southwark, London.* London: MoLAS Monograph 3.

Brown, R. 1986. *The English Baptists of the 18th Century.* London: The Baptist Historical Society.

Cross, F.L. and Livingstone, E.A. (eds.) 1997. *The Oxford Dictionary of the Christian Church.* Oxford: Oxford University Press.

Davies, G.J. 1994. "Poole shipping in the eighteenth century" *Proceedings of the Dorset Natural History and Archaeological Society* 116: 21-25.

Densham, W. and Ogle, J. (eds.) 1899. *The Story of the Congregational Churches of Dorset, from their Foundation to the Present Time.* Bournemouth: W. Mate & Son.

Doel, W. 1890. *Twenty Golden Candlesticks... a History of Baptist Nonconformity in Western Wiltshire.* Trowbridge: Trowbridge.

Gilchrist, R. and Sloane, B. 2005. *Requiem. The medieval monastic cemetery in Britain.* London: MoLAS.

Hutchins, J. 1803. *The History and Antiquities of the County of Dorset: Volume 2.* London: J. Nichols.

Hutchins, J. 1861 *The History and Antiquities of the County of Dorset: Volume 1.* London: Bowyer and Nichols.

Johnson, S. and McKinley, J.I. forthcoming. "Nonconformity and Baptists in 18th century Poole" In: McKinley, J.I. *The 18th Century Baptist Chapel and Burial Ground at West Butts Street, Poole.* Salisbury: Wessex Archaeology Report No. 21.

Legg, R. 2005. *The Book of Poole. Harbour and Town.* Tiverton: Halsgrove.

Lewis, M.E. 2007 *The Bioarchaeology of Children. Perspectives from Biological and Forensic Anthropology* Cambridge: Cambridge University Press.

Mahoney, D. 2005. "Quaker inhumations". In: Brown, R. *Vancouver Centre and Clough Lane Car Park, King's Lynn, Norfolk. Post excavation Assessment and Updated Project Design.* Oxford Archaeology (unpublished).

McKee, A. 1974. "The influence of British Navy strategy on ship design: 1400-1850". In: Bass, G.F. (ed.) *A History of Seafaring, Based on Underwater Archaeology* London: Thames and Hudson. 226-252.

McKinley, J.I. forthcoming. "The People". In: McKinley, J.I. *The 18th Century Baptist Chapel and Burial Ground at West Butts Street, Poole.* Salisbury: Wessex Archaeology Report No. 21.

McKinley, J.I. and Egging, K. forthcoming. "The Excavations". In: McKinley, J.I. *The 18th Century Baptist Chapel and Burial Ground at West Butts Street, Poole.* Salisbury: Wessex Archaeology Report No. 21.

Medlycott, M. 1999. *Index to Dorset Militia Ballot Lists 1757-1799. Volume 1 – East Dorset.* Weymouth: Somerset and Dorset Family History Society.

Mepham, L. and Every, R. forthcoming. "The metalwork". In: McKinley, J.I. *The 18th Century Baptist*

Chapel and Burial Ground at West Butts Street, Poole. Salisbury: Wessex Archaeology Report No. 21.

Molleson, T. and Cox, M. 1993. *The Spitalfields Project. Volume 2: the anthropology. The Middling Sort.* York: Council for British Archaeology Research Report 86.

Penn, K.J. 1980. *Historic Towns in Dorset*, Dortchester: Dorset Natural History and Archaeological Society Monograph No. 1.

Roberts, C. and Cox, M. 2003 *Health and Disease in Britain from Prehistory to the Present Day.* Stroud: Sutton.

Scheuer, L. 1998. "Age at death and cause of death of the people buried at St. Bride's Church, Fleet Street, London". In: Cox, M. (ed.) *Grave Concerns. Death and burials in England 1700-1850.* York: Council for British Archaeology Research Report 113. 100-111.

Short, B.C. 1927. *Early Days of Nonconformity in Poole.* Poole: J. Looker.

Smith, H.P. 1948. *The History of the Borough and County of the Town of Poole Vol. 1: Origins and early development.* Poole: Looker.

Smith, H.P. 1951. *The History of the Borough and County of the Town of Poole Vol. 2: County Corporate Status.* Poole: Looker.

Sydenham, J. 1839. *The History of Poole.* (1986 facsimile edition) Poole: Poole Historic Trust.

Walker, J.B. 1981. "The children in the cemetery: child mortality and public health in Lyme Regis 1856 to 1979" *Proceedings of the Dorset Natural History and Archaeological Society* 103: 5-12.

www.ingramcontent.com/pod-product-compliance
Lightning Source LLC
Chambersburg PA
CBHW061003030426
42334CB00033B/3346